The Weight
Training
HANDBOOK

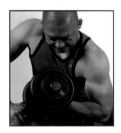

Wayne Viljoen

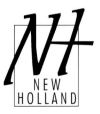

NEW
HOLLAND

The Weight
Training
HANDBOOK

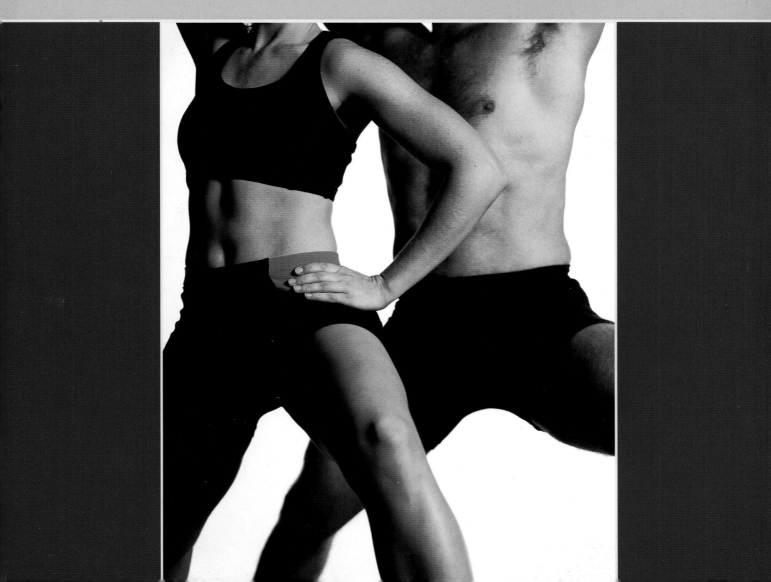

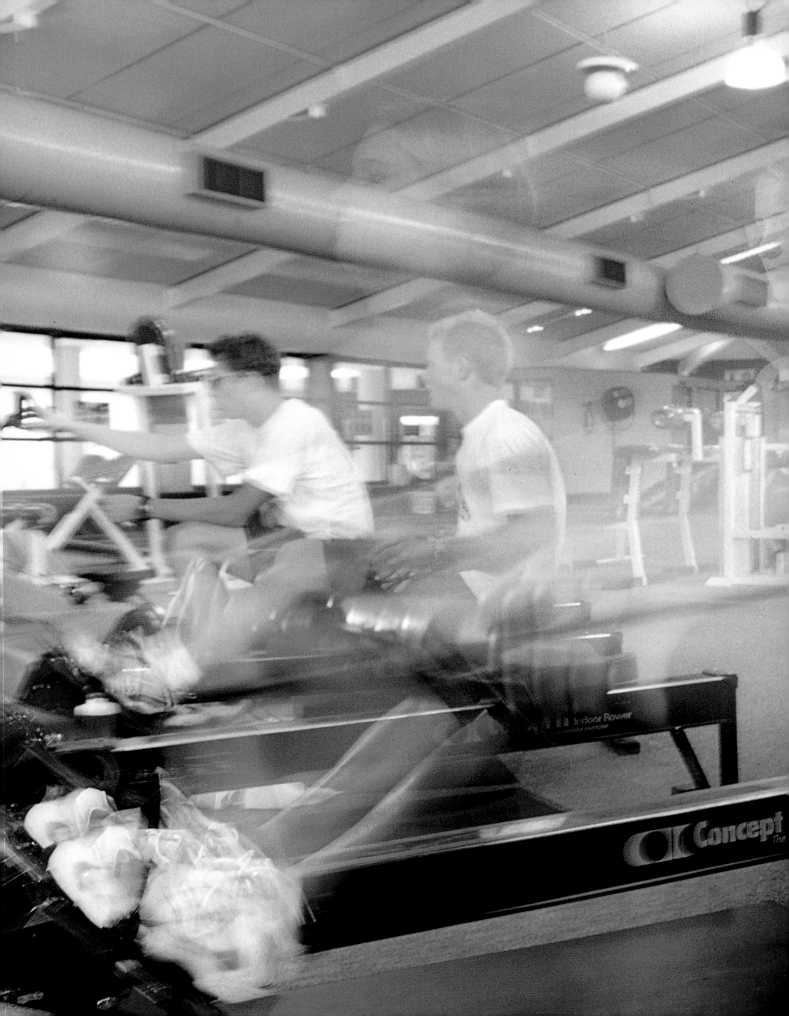

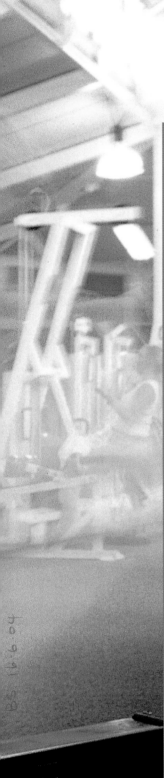
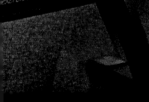

First published in 2003 by New Holland Publishers

London • Cape Town • Sydney • Auckland

www.newhollandpublishers.com

86 Edgware Road	14 Aquatic Drive	80 McKenzie Street	218 Lake Road
London	Frenchs Forest	Cape Town	Northcote
W2 2EA	NSW 2086	8001	Auckland
United Kingdom	Australia	South Africa	New Zealand

ISBN 1 84330 349 3 (HB)

ISBN 1 84330 350 7 (PB)

Reproduction by Hirt & Carter (Cape) Pty Ltd

Printed and bound in Malaysia by Times Offset (M) Sdn. Bhd

10 9 8 7 6 5 4 3 2 1

Although the publishers have made every effort to ensure that the information contained
in this book was meticulously researched and correct at the time of going to press,
they accept no responsibility for any inaccuracies, loss, injury or inconvenience
sustained by any person using this book.

PUBLISHER	Mariëlle Renssen	DESIGN CONCEPT	Christelle Marais
PUBLISHING MANAGERS	Claudia dos Santos,	DESIGNER	Damian Gibbs
	Simon Pooley	ILLUSTRATOR	Steven Felmore
COMMISSIONING EDITOR	Alfred LeMaitre	PRODUCTION	Myrna Collins
MANAGING ART EDITOR	Richard MacArthur	PROOFREADER	Mariëlle Renssen
EDITOR	Anna Tanneberger	INDEXER	Leizel Brown

CONSULTANT Dr Nick Walters, Vice Principal British College of Osteopathic Medicine

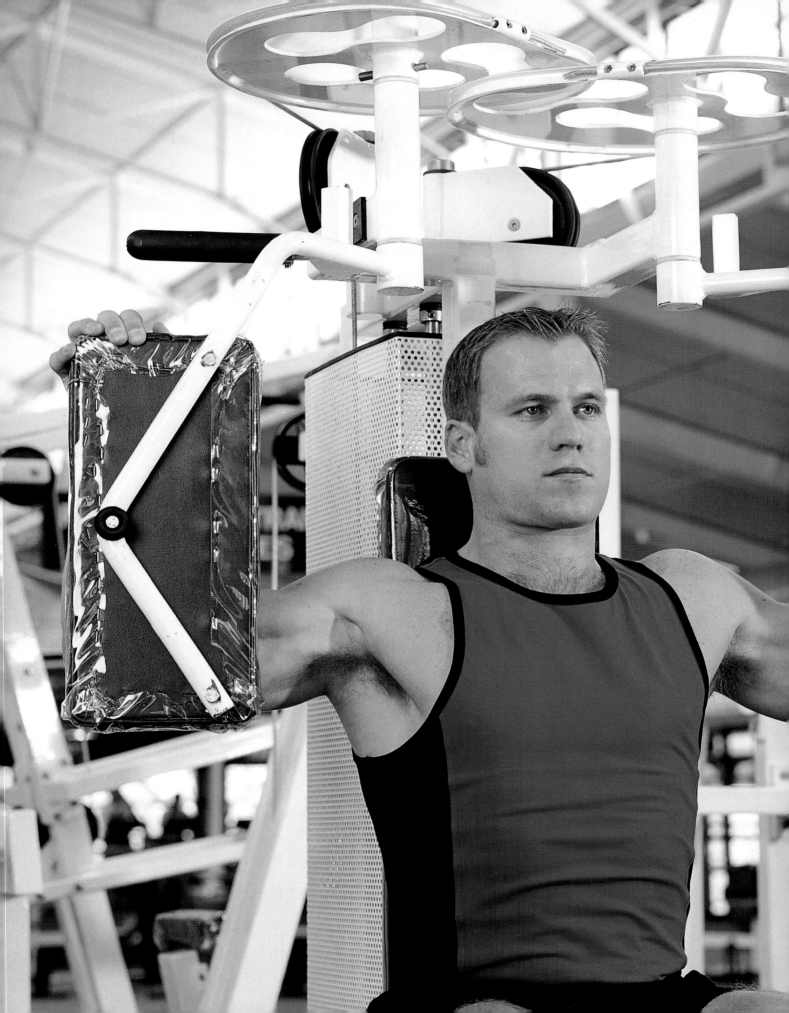

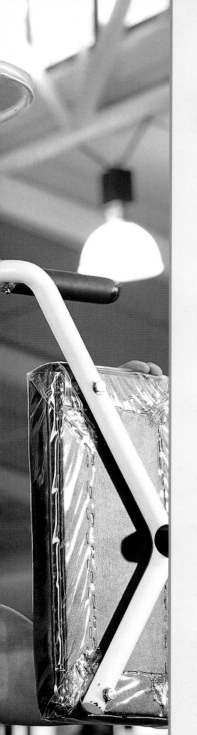

Contents

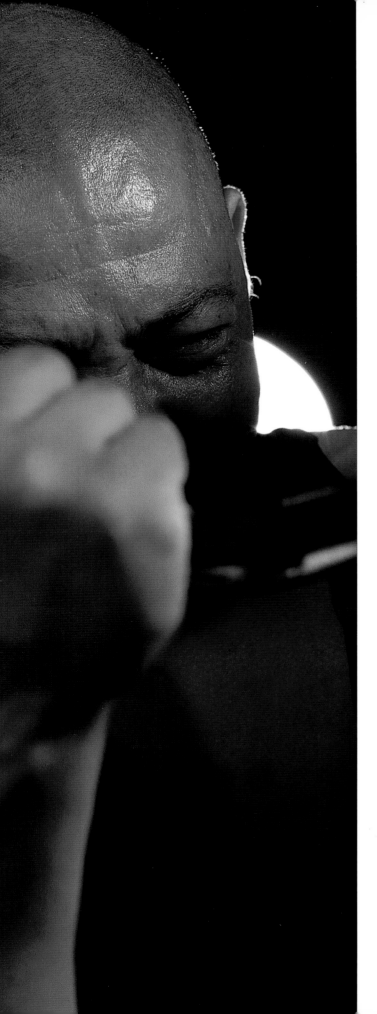

Introduction to weight training

The emergence of the technological era has resulted in a shift towards a sedentary lifestyle. This has given rise to an increase in the prevalence of chronic diseases such as obesity and diabetes. Most people now realize that exercise is the best way to ward off the onset of these conditions.

Health clubs and gyms have become popular and weight, strength and resistance training have become household names.

What is weight training?

Weight training (resistance training) involves moving (or attempting to move) a weight; or moving against a resistive force through a range of motion. This resistive force can be presented in the form of machine equipment, free weights or even your own body weight. Another form of resistance training is aqua aerobics, which involves moving against the resistance of water. In elastic-band exercises, such as with Theraband and surgical tubing, resistance increases exponentially as the band or tubing is stretched. Calisthenics uses your own body weight as resistance, for example, when you do push-ups.

Most exercise routines involve the use of free weights or standard machines. Free weights consist of barbells and dumbbells. Machines use various methods to load the muscles, such as a cable-and-pulley system, free weights, or a cam which changes the effective load during movement (dynamic variable-resistance machine).

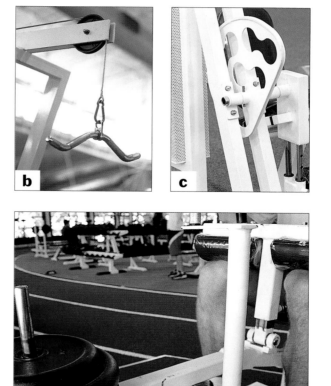

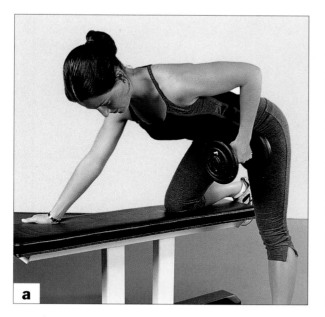

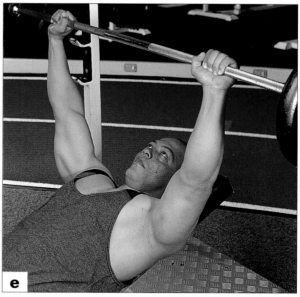

(a) A free weight exercise with a dumbbell. (b) A cable attached to a weight-stack and handle. The cable is directed along pulleys to apply a resistive force. (c) The cam of a dynamic variable-resistance machine varies the resistance during movement. (d) Free-weight machines, such as this calf-raise machine, load the muscles with weight plates stacked onto the equipment. (e) A free-weight exercise performed using a barbell.

The benefits of resistance training

Most people associate resistance training with Olympic weightlifters, power lifters and bodybuilders. However, anyone can benefit from resistance training. In fact, the room for improvement in muscle strength, endurance and body composition (increased muscle mass and loss of body fat) is far greater in relatively unfit individuals than in trained athletes.

Training goals

A major misconception about resistance training is that it only involves the use of heavy, maximal weights – the maximum weight a person can lift through one repetition. Many women fear they will end up looking like The Incredible Hulk. This is far from the truth. Resistance training entails the use of weights, or resistance, to achieve goals such as gaining or losing weight, toning and firming muscle, and improving cardiovascular endurance and muscle strength.

Your body composition, current training status and fitness-test results will determine which training programme level – beginner, intermediate or advanced – will benefit you most.

Somatotyping

One factor that will have a big influence on the selection of your training goal is your body shape. Another name for this is somatotyping, which categorizes your body into degrees of body-fat

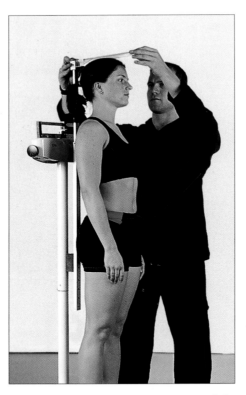

Standing height is an important measure in body composition assessment. It is used to calculate body mass index, and to determine muscularity and leanness. It is important to remember that these are all relative measures.

content, musculoskeletal development and leanness. The main body shapes are primary endomorph, mesomorph and ectomorph, which refer to individuals who are predominantly fat, muscular or lean.

There are also combinations of these primary body shapes. An endo-mesomorph, for example, is predominantly muscular, but with a tendency to have excess body fat. A meso-ectomorph would be predominantly lean, but with a tendency to be quite muscular.

For the purpose of somatotyping, you will need to know your body composition. This can be calculated by taking skinfold measurements and using a formula based on the theory that subcutaneous fat (under the skin) makes up 50% of your total body-fat count. Your muscular and bone development should be determined by means of bone diameter and muscle circumference measurements. Your degree of leanness can be measured by using an index based on your height and body mass.

Assessing body composition

Lean body mass consists of muscle, bone and residual mass – fluid, tissue and organs – and can be determined once your total body fat has been calculated. Various techniques of estimating total body fat have evolved over the years, including skinfold measurement, infrared scanning, bioelectrical impedance, hydrostatic (underwater) weighing, dual-energy X-ray absorptiometry (DEXA), and air displacement plethysmography. The latter three are the most accurate, with a measurement error of less than 2%. By comparison, the other techniques can have a measurement error of up to 8–10%. Unfortunately, the most accurate techniques are also the most expensive. The most affordable and most frequently used method is skinfold measurement. The disadvantage of this method is that various different equations are used to calculate body fat, making it difficult to assess progress when comparing measurements taken by different professionals at different institutions. The kind of calliper used and the individual skill of the tester also affect the reliability of this method. When measuring extremely obese individuals, the callipers cannot pinch all their skinfolds at the required sites. Nevertheless, it can be a useful gauge of body composition.

Another indirect, and inexpensive, method of checking your body type is by calculating your body mass index (BMI). This is done by measuring your body mass and dividing it by your standing height in metres squared. This gives a ratio of body mass to height in kg/m². For example:

$84kg \ divided \ by \ (1.78m)^2 = 26.5 \ kg/m^2$

This ratio negates your physical size and can provide significant information on whether you are underweight, average, overweight or obese. However, it measures muscularity as much as fatness. For that reason body mass index is not relevant for people such as athletes or top sportsmen.

When you are tested by a fitness professional using a specific technique, you should monitor your progress at regular

TABLE OF BMI CLASSIFICATION: WORLD HEALTH ORGANIZATION CLASSIFICATION OF OBESITY

Classification	BMI	Risk of co-morbidity
Underweight	<18.5	Low
Normal weight	18.5–25	Average
Overweight	25–29.9	Increased
Obese Class 1	29.9–34.9	Moderate
Obese Class 2	34.9–39.9	Severe
Obese Class 3	>39.9	Very severe

intervals by returning to the same tester, using the same technique. This ensures consistency, which will give you a useful comparison of your current body composition to your previous status.

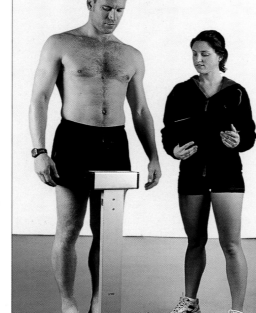

Body mass measurements can be used to monitor weight-gain (hypertrophy), weight-loss and weight-maintenance programmes.

Needs analysis

As part of your assessment by a professional you will need a complete health and activity analysis as well as a fitness and training goal assessment. This usually includes a body composition analysis.

Fitness professionals use many screening tools to help them identify their clients' needs and, of course, a fitness test would help. However, the most suitable programme for you is determined by what you want to achieve. Remember, good training results do not come easily, so dig deep. It is not the destination, but the journey that matters.

COMPARISON OF RESULTS OF BODY COMPOSITION DETERMINED WITH DIFFERENT FORMULAE

Different formulae were used to assess a 31-year-old male weighing 84kg (185lb) and 1.78m (5ft 10in) tall.

Skinfold-sites	Values (mm)	% Body fat using the formulae of Drinkwater and Ross	% Body fat using the formulae of Heath-Carter	% Body fat using the formulae of Durnin and Womersley	Sum of skinfolds method of Ross and Marfell-Jones
Triceps	10.0	9.08%	13.8%	16.3%	63.6mm
Subscapular	8.9	Normative range for this person	Normative range for this person	Normative range for this person	Normative range for sedentary individuals
Supra-iliac	8.1	(10-12%)	(12-15%)	(14-16%)	(120mm)
Biceps	3.5				
Calf	7.0				
Abdominal	12.6				
Thigh	13.5				

Measurement of (a) calf muscle circumference, (b) forearm circumference, (c) humerus bone diameter, (d) femur bone diameter, and (e) contracted biceps circumference. Skinfold measurement sites: (f) triceps, (g) subscapular, (h) medial calf, (i) mid-thigh, (j) abdomen, (k) supra-iliac, and (l) biceps.

Basic dietary recommendations

Your main contributing energy source during resistance training is **carbohydrates**, and this needs to be replaced after training. The majority (55–60%) of your daily caloric intake should be carbohydrates such as sugars, fruits, pastas and breads. Endurance athletes generally require higher intakes. Carbohydrate drinks and supplements taken after exercise may assist recovery, limit protein breakdown and benefit your immune system.

Protein should constitute about 15–20% of your daily caloric intake. Preferred sources are from animal proteins such as eggs, dairy products and meat. Corn, nuts, legumes and grains are also sources of protein. When you are training heavily, the maximum amount of protein you need is about 1.5–2 gram per kilogram of body mass (g/kg) or 0.0015 to 0.002 per cent of your body mass. This is higher than the normal daily requirement of 0.8–1g/kg. Many protein and 'mass building' shakes recommend more than 4g/kg servings, which just ends up as expensive urine because your body simply excretes the excess.

When in need of more specific advice and an appropriate diet, it is better to consult a qualified sport nutritionist or registered dietician. A well-balanced diet should provide sufficient protein and carbohydrates for your requirements, so that there is very little need to buy expensive nutritional supplements.

Something all newcomers will come across in the gym sooner or later is **steroids**. Anabolic steroids have special medical uses and are often prescribed for certain muscle-wasting diseases and for males with very low levels of naturally produced testosterone and impotence. In gyms they are sometimes abused by healthy people looking for quick results in increasing muscle mass, improving strength, reducing the muscle breakdown and enhancing recovery. However, there is no shortcut to success. If you climb the ladder too quickly there is a good chance you will fall off! Numerous side effects have been associated with steroid abuse. In males it has been associated with acne, infertility, shrinking testes, development of breasts (gynaecomastia) and prostate cancer. In females it may lead to baldness, a deeper voice, increased body hair and facial hair. Other side effects are liver cancer, increases in LDL ('bad') cholesterol, decreases in HDL ('good') cholesterol, aggression and addiction to name but a few. Avoid the seductive trap of quick results. The risks associated with the abuse of anabolic steroids significantly outweigh any benefits that might accrue in using them.

DYNAMIC VARIABLE RESISTANCE MACHINES

When training with free weights, standard cable pulley machines and the majority of free weight machines, the resistance supplied remains more or less constant throughout the range of motion of the exercise. However, at some point during the execution of an exercise, there is a change in leverage due to a change in position, reducing the mechanical advantage of the muscle being used. The amount of resistance that can be shifted past this sticking point is therefore the maximum load that can be used in this exercise. This type of resistance training is called 'dynamic constant external resistance' exercise.

This limit can be overcome by dynamic variable resistance machines, which use a cam device to vary the amount of resistance applied according to the changes in leverage during the execution of the exercise. This adjustment increases the load that can be used to train that body part, muscle or muscle group. The cam of a dynamic variable-resistance machine is illustrated in photograph (c) on page 9.

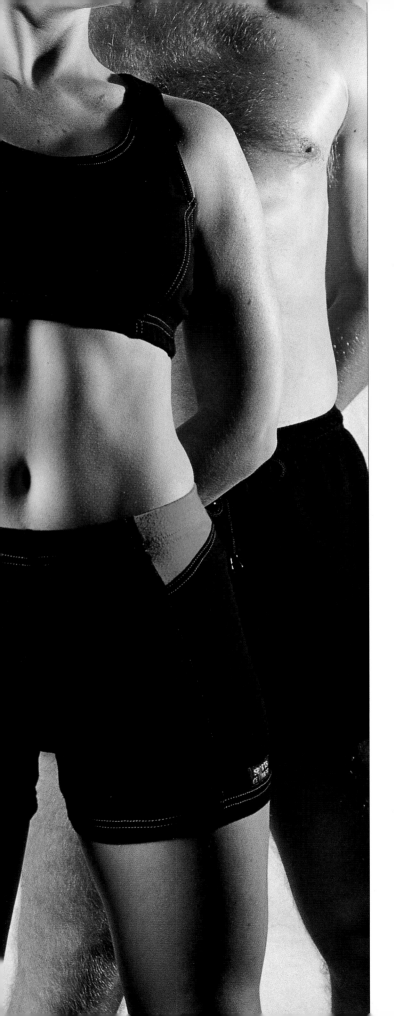

Basic anatomy and physiology

Two of the most important components of the human body in terms of weight training are muscle and bone. They hold you together and upright, allow you to move from point A to point B and prevent you from falling apart! Muscle also stabilizes joints, generates body heat and maintains posture.

There are three types of muscle: cardiac, smooth, and skeletal muscle.

Cardiac muscle

Cardiac muscle is only found in the heart and makes up the majority of the heart wall mass. It is also called involuntary muscle, because we have no conscious control of it. The heart's pacemaker, or sino-atrial node, controls the rate at which it contracts.

Smooth muscle

Smooth muscle is also an involuntary muscle. It is found in the walls of various organs and vessels, such as in the oesophageal wall which reflexively contracts and relaxes in an action called peristalsis, enabling us to swallow.

Skeletal muscle

Skeletal muscles are classified as voluntary muscles and are the longest of the three muscle types. However,

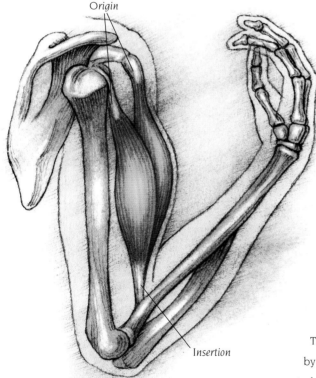

Origin

Insertion

The origin and insertion of the biceps brachii. Movement occurs when the insertion is pulled towards the origin.

despite being voluntary, they are also regulated by involuntary reflexes. This reflex mechanism also has a significant impact on particular training techniques. Skeletal muscle is generally powerful and fatigues quite easily compared to other muscle types. It must therefore be rested regularly, a factor that has to be taken into account in planning training programmes.

Movement

In any movement, a muscle must bring two or more bones together. Muscle must be connected to bone; the relevant terms used here are: muscle origin (where the muscle starts) and muscle insertion (where it stops). The bone at which the muscle originates does not move, or moves little, when that muscle contracts. The bone at the other end of the muscle generally moves towards the origin when the muscle contracts. The insertion is usually located further away from the torso. For example, the biceps' muscle origin is at the shoulder and its insertion at the forearm.

A skeletal muscle is made up of hundreds of muscle fibres, numerous blood vessels, nerve connections and connective tissue. However, without a structure that organizes and controls the muscle and body parts, and without a binding structure that connects the muscle to bone, and bone to bone, movement would not occur. Hence the importance of the nervous system and connective tissue structures in the body.

The nervous system

The main function of muscle is to produce movement by contracting and relaxing. It is controlled by the central nervous system to achieve smooth and coordinated movements. The **central nervous system** (brain, brain stem and spinal cord) controls, coordinates, processes and regulates all incoming and outgoing information. The **peripheral nervous system** (sensory and motor nerves) relays all the information between the central nervous system and the muscles and organs. It is also responsible for various involuntary spinal reflexes. Without the central and peripheral nervous systems working together, movement would be erratic and uncontrolled.

Connective tissue

Connective tissue is important in resistance training programmes because of its integral role in the transfer of muscle force to bone (via tendons) and in efficient movement by stabilizing the joint and preventing excessive or unwanted motion (via ligaments). A tendon is an example of predominantly collagenous connective tissue that connects muscle to bone. It is a rigid structure that can only stretch to about 5% of its resting length and, by transferring the forces generated by active muscle to bone, it contributes to movement by pulling the bones towards each other.

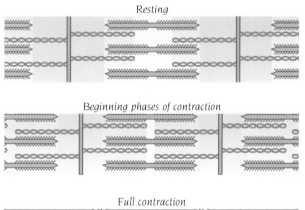

Resting

Beginning phases of contraction

Full contraction

━━ Z-disk ⊞⊞⊞ Myosin ⋈⊙⊙⊙ Actin

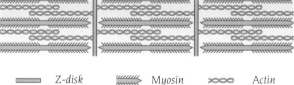

Shortening of the sarcomere (muscle's contractile unit) occurs when the actin myofilaments are pulled over the myosin filaments by means of cross-bridge cycling.

Muscle structure

A muscle consists of thousands of muscle cells or muscle fibres. Each of these muscle fibres is surrounded by connective tissue that is continuous with the muscle membrane (sarcolemma). This keeps the cells, which are generally fragile and soft, together. This connective tissue sheath is called the endomysium. Numerous encapsulated muscle fibres are bundled together into fascicles (bundles), which are covered by a further layer of collagenous connective tissue called the perimysium. To further strengthen the integrity of muscle, the groups of fascicles are ensheathed by an even stronger layer of connective tissue called the epimysium, which surrounds the entire muscle. These various layers of connective tissue link all the individual muscle fibres, are themselves interconnected and terminate in the respective tendinous origins and insertions of the muscle.

The tendons insert into another type of connective tissue structure called the periosteum, consisting of double-layered tissue covering all the bones in the body. When an individual fibre contracts, the force generated by that muscle fibre is summated with each of the other contracting fibres and transferred by the connective tissue structures to the bones. The bones are then pulled towards each other to create movement.

How do skeletal muscles contract?

Having established that each muscle is comprised of numerous fibres, each of these in turn consists of many myofibrils, which form the functional units of muscle and effect the contraction and relaxation process. The functional part of the myofibrils consists of numerous contractile units, called sarcomeres, connected in series. Each sarcomere is composed of different muscle proteins, in particular the two main contractile proteins (myofilaments) called actin and myosin. Myosin filaments are thick contractile proteins and remain relatively stationary during contraction. Actin filaments

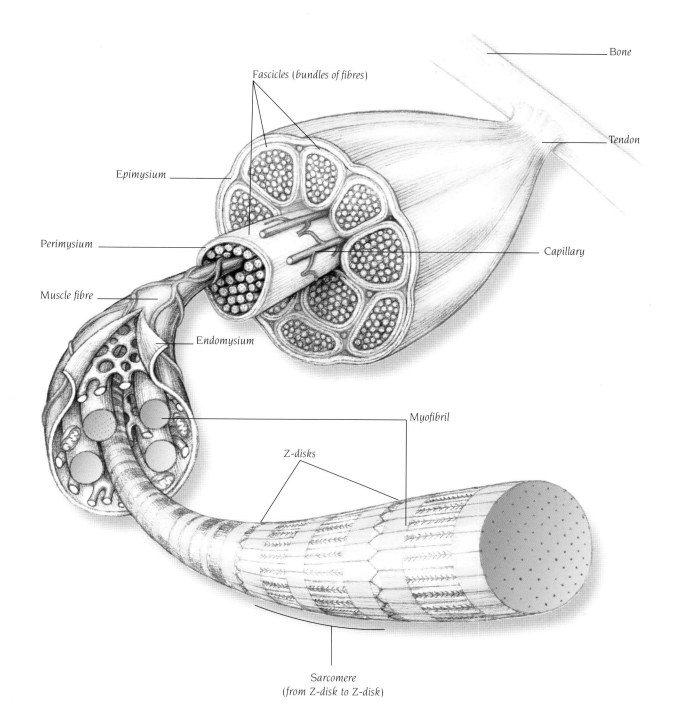

Bone

Tendon

Fascicles (bundles of fibres)

Epimysium

Perimysium

Capillary

Muscle fibre

Endomysium

Myofibril

Z-disks

Sarcomere
(from Z-disk to Z-disk)

The substructure of a muscle. A muscle is made up of collective bundles of muscle fibres. These consist of numerous myofibrils composed mainly of the contractile proteins actin and myosin, which are responsible for effecting muscle contraction. The forces generated by the muscle fibres are transferred via various interconnected connective tissue structures to the tendinous origin and insertion of the muscle-tendon complex to create or resist movement.

are thin contractile proteins that are drawn towards each other from both ends of the sarcomere during muscle contraction. The actin and myosin filaments lie parallel to each other and become interlocked during contraction. The two contractile proteins are connected during contraction by myosin cross-bridges. (These are globular proteins that originate from the larger myosin filaments and are chemically bound to the actin filaments during contraction.)

When contracting, the actin myofilaments from both ends of the sarcomere slide over the myosin filaments towards the middle of the sarcomere, thereby shortening the contractile unit by pulling the Z-disks towards each other. This is similar to the forward movement of a millipede. The cross-bridges attach and detach in different sequences (the way a millipede's legs move along the ground) to pull the actin filaments over the myosin filaments. Not all myosin cross-bridges are attached at the same time.

The difference between the millipede and cross-bridges is that the cross-bridge cycling is significantly faster. As each sarcomere shortens, the entire muscle fibre contracts. Depending on how many myofibrils are activated, their respective forces are also summated and transferred by the tendons and tendinous structures to the bones.

Different forms of muscle contraction

Most people associate muscle contraction with muscle shortening and a decreasing angle between two bones. However, it also means that the muscle attempts to shorten against, or actively resists while lengthening against, a load. To avoid this misunderstanding, many exercise scientists and fitness professionals use the term 'muscle action' to describe how muscles function, but I still prefer to use the term 'muscle contraction'.

There are four different types of muscle contraction, namely • concentric • eccentric • isometric • plyometric.

CONCENTRIC CONTRACTION

The most common muscle contractions in resistance training are concentric and eccentric. Concentric contraction means that the muscle is activating sufficient myosin-actin cross-bridges to develop enough muscle tension to overcome the load or weights applied upon it. The muscle therefore shortens and closes the joint angle between two bones by pulling the insertion of the muscle towards its origin. In other words, the muscle generates sufficient force to overcome and lift the weight. This is also known as a positive contraction. The lifting phase of resistance training is a concentric contraction. For most concentric contractions, the duration of the contraction should be roughly one to two seconds from beginning to end. This is not, however, true for all techniques.

ECCENTRIC CONTRACTION

Once the weight has been lifted, it has to be lowered to its starting position. This must be done in a controlled manner – for safety reasons as well as for training benefits. While the muscle lengthens and prevents the weights from falling down, the muscle is contracting eccentrically and resists lengthening. The lowering phase of resistance training is an eccentric contraction. Eccentric contractions should last roughly two to four seconds from beginning to end, though not for all techniques.

ISOMETRIC CONTRACTION

Isometric contraction is often defined as 'muscle contraction without muscle shortening and without visible movement' although the muscle does shorten to some extent as it contracts against the opposing tendons of the origin and insertion. In this way it applies tension to them and the tendinous structures, and statically supports a submaximal load (less than the maximum load you can lift), or tries to overcome a supramaximal load (more than you can lift). The resistance used, and compliance of the tendons, determine the extent to which the tendons can stretch and the muscles shorten. A better definition would be 'a static muscle contraction where no movement of the

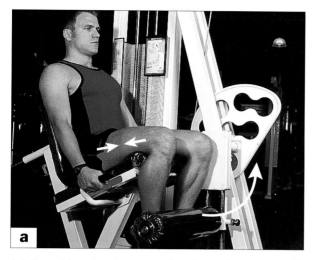

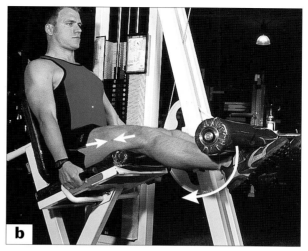

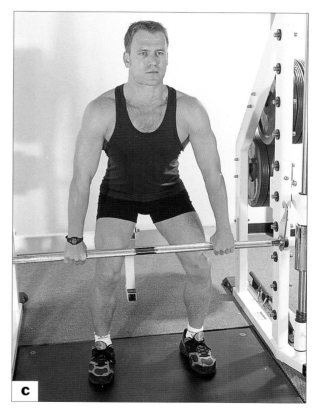

(*a*) *Concentric contraction occurs when the muscles generate sufficient force to overcome inertia and lift the weight. Arrows show the direction of movement and of muscle pull.*

(*b*) *Eccentric contraction occurs when the weights are lowered (the muscles resist lengthening).*

(*c*) *In an isometric contraction no movement is visible, while the muscles try to overcome an immovable load or hold a submaximal load in a static position. Here the top stoppers resist movement.*

limb or body part involved is visible'. In other words, an isometric contraction is a static contraction, where the muscle's tendinous insertion and origin do not approach each other, even though the muscle sarcomeres shorten slightly to support or attempt to move the load. Holding a lighter weight stationary, and trying to lift an immovable object are examples of isometric contractions.

PLYOMETRIC MUSCLE ACTION

Plyometric muscle action is the stretch-shortening cycle of a muscle. In this instance I prefer the term muscle action to contraction because plyometric action features the combination of eccentric and concentric contractions when a load is lifted. Most natural and sporting movements make use of the stretch-shortening cycle. In any sporting movement, if you intend to move in one direction, you unconsciously move in the opposite direction first and prestretch the muscle before pushing off in the intended direction. A side step in rugby or football is a

good example. The term stretch-shortening cycle perfectly describes it: first you stretch the muscle and then you shorten it. You use a quick eccentric stretch of the involved muscle to enhance the concentric contraction to follow. In resistance training, this is a fast and explosive technique used for developing explosiveness and power.

THE MAIN MUSCLE GROUPS OF THE BODY

To make more sense of resistance-training programmes and techniques, you need to know the main muscle groups of the body. There are more than 600 muscles in the body, but I've included only the major ones of functional importance to resistance training.

The main large muscle groups of the body are:

- Chest (pectoralis major, pectoralis minor, serratus anterior, intercostalis).
- Upper arms (biceps brachii, brachialis, triceps brachii).
- Shoulders (anterior, posterior and middle deltoid, infraspinatus, supraspinatus, teres major).
- Upper back (latissimus dorsi, rhomboid major, and trapezius).
- Thigh, which consists of the hamstrings (biceps femoris, semimembranosus and semitendinosus); the

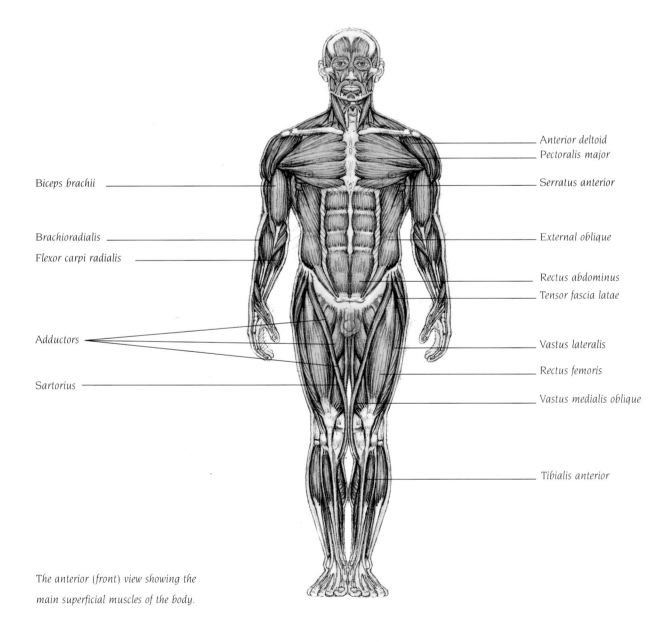

Biceps brachii

Brachioradialis

Flexor carpi radialis

Adductors

Sartorius

Anterior deltoid
Pectoralis major

Serratus anterior

External oblique

Rectus abdominus
Tensor fascia latae

Vastus lateralis

Rectus femoris

Vastus medialis oblique

Tibialis anterior

The anterior (front) view showing the main superficial muscles of the body.

quadriceps (rectus femoris, vastus medialis oblique and vastus lateralis); the adductor group (adductor magnus and adductor longus); gracilis; sartorius; and tensor fascia latae.

- Abdomen (rectus abdominus, transverse abdominus, internal and external oblique).

Smaller muscle groups:

- Forearms (brachioradialis, pronator teres, flexor carpi radialis, palmaris longus, flexor carpi ulnaris, extensor carpi radialis longus, extensor carpi ulnaris).
- Lower back (erector spinae, quadratus lumborum, multifidus).
- Hip (iliopsoas, pectineus, gluteus maximus, gluteus medius, tensor fascia latae).
- Lower leg (soleus, gastrocnemius, peroneus longus, extensor digitorum longus, tibialis anterior).

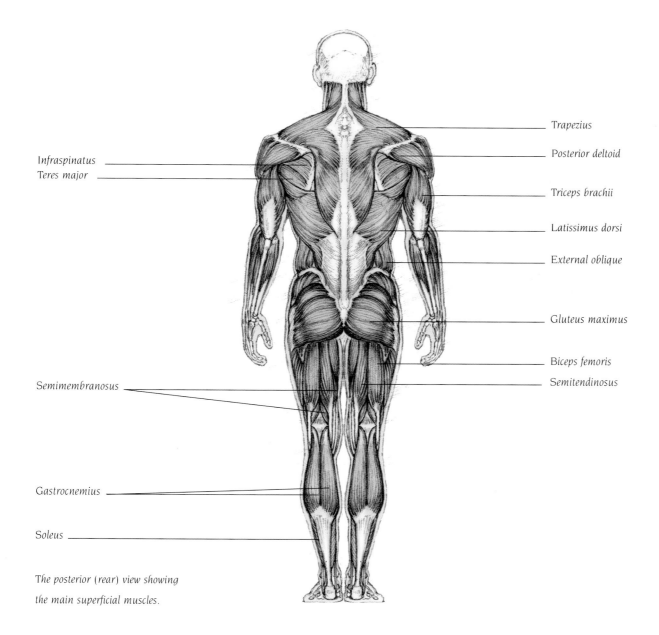

Infraspinatus
Teres major

Semimembranosus

Gastrocnemius

Soleus

Trapezius

Posterior deltoid

Triceps brachii

Latissimus dorsi

External oblique

Gluteus maximus

Biceps femoris

Semitendinosus

The posterior (rear) view showing the main superficial muscles.

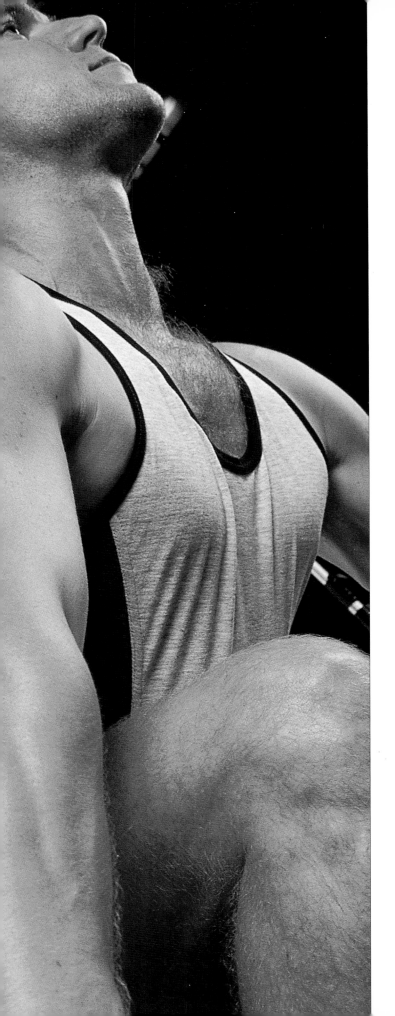

Correct training

Because of the nature of resistance training, you need to prepare your body for action in order to decrease the risk of injury. This is done through a progressive warm-up, starting with generalized aerobic activity, through to stretches specific to the muscle groups to be trained in the main workout. One major concern with regards to weight training is that it can be dangerous if performed incorrectly. This chapter will give basic guidelines on the fundamentals, accessories and safety considerations.

General warm-up

The body needs to be warmed up with some low-intensity aerobic activity such as jogging, cycling, rope skipping, rowing or stair climbing for 5–10 minutes. The intensity of the general warm-up should be just enough to cause you to break into a light sweat. The purpose of the general warm-up is to increase blood flow to the working muscles and to elevate the body's core temperature. This helps muscles to contract and relax quickly and easily. The extensibility of connective tissue is enhanced, reducing the risk of injury. Neural mechanisms and responses are improved, facilitating efficient, controlled movements.

Specific warm-up

Follow the aerobic warm-up with a series of static and dynamic stretches. Stretching cold muscles can injure them. Hold each static stretch for 20–30 seconds and repeat once or twice. Perform this routine as part of a warm-up and, if possible, afterwards as part of the cool-down. This helps prevent injury and improves recovery after an intense workout.

The following general stretch routine covers most of the body and is suitable for any programme. Stretching should not be painful. You should feel the muscle pulling taut, but no pain. Stretch slowly and do not bounce. Inhale deeply before, and exhale into, each stretch.

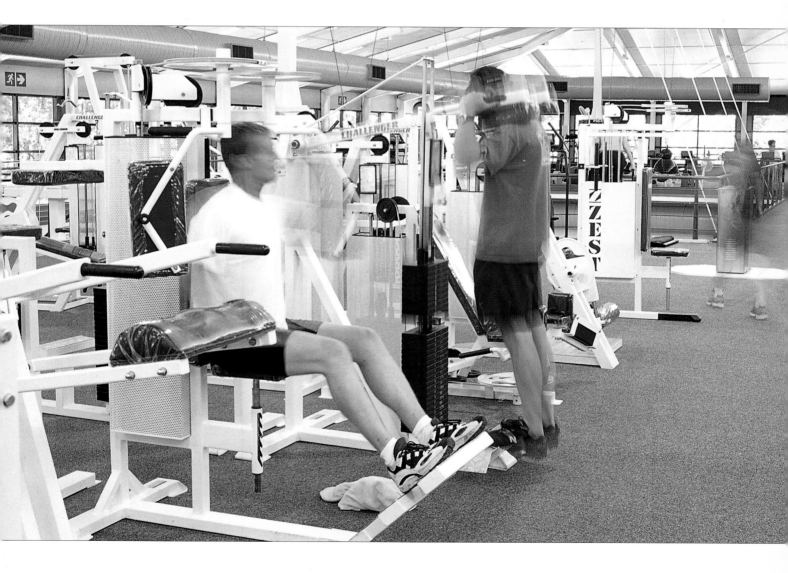

Stretches

Chest and anterior shoulders

▶ **Stretch 1:** Stand upright, with your right shoulder to the wall. Place the palm of your right hand against the wall at about shoulder level, with your shoulder abducted – upper arm lifted away from the centreline of the body (*see glossary p122*) – and arm flexed at 45°. While keeping the palm of your hand against the wall and flexed elbow pointing downward, exhale and move forward slightly with your left leg. Slowly turn your body away from the fixed hand and the wall, until the front of your shoulder muscle and chest are pulled taut. Hold the stretch, and relax back to the starting position. Swap sides and hands, and repeat the stretch on the other side.

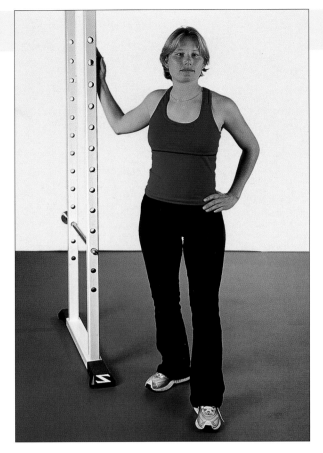

See glossary, p122, for terms such as adduction, abduction and anatomical position.

▼ **Stretch 2:** Sit upright with your arms extended behind you, hands on the ground, fingers pointing away from the body, palms down. Exhale, lean back and slide the buttocks forward while maintaining the hand position. Hold the stretch, relax and repeat.

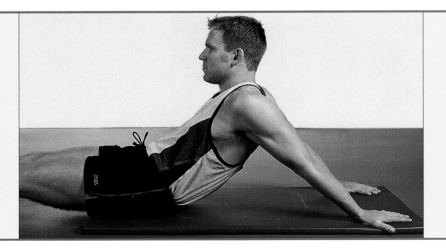

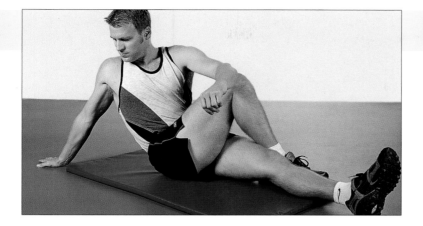
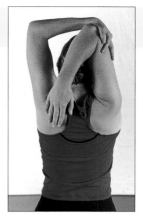

Lower back, torso and hips

▲ **Stretch 3:** This is a compound stretch. Sit with your left leg extended in front of you and the right arm extended behind you on the ground. Interlock your right leg over your left leg with the knee flexed and the foot on the ground. Move the right foot as close as possible towards the left buttock, so that the right knee approaches the chest. Use the left arm to pull the knee closer if necessary. Twist the torso to the right and place the left elbow outside the right knee, while keeping the right arm extended behind you. Once in this position, continue to twist the torso to the right and pull the right knee towards the chest with the left elbow. Hold the stretch and relax. Repeat on the other side.

Upper arms ▲

Stretch 4: Stand upright with your right upper arm raised, pressing against your right ear, and elbow flexed with the right hand hanging over your left shoulder blade. Place your left hand on your right elbow. Exhale, and with the left hand, pull the elbow further down behind the head. Hold the stretch and relax. Repeat on the other side.

Upper back and posterior shoulders

▼ **Stretch 5:** Stand with your right arm extended and raised to shoulder height, and your thumb facing up. Horizontally adduct the straight arm across your chest by slowly swinging it across from the right to the left side of your body with your upper arm passing underneath your chin. Exhale and, using the left hand, pull the extended arm towards the neck. Hold, relax and repeat on the other side.

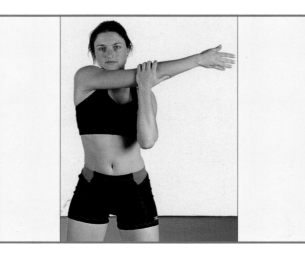

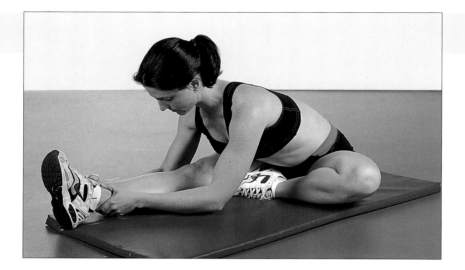

Lower back and hamstrings

▲ **Stretch 6:** Sit upright with the right leg extended in front of you, the left leg flexed and the left foot pressed against the inner thigh of the right leg. Bend the right knee slightly. Grasp the right leg with both hands, as close as possible to the ankle. Do not overestimate your ability. If you can only grasp the calf muscle, that is fine. Keep both hands at the same level and have the chest facing the right leg. Once you have grasped the right leg, extend or straighten the right knee. Exhale and move the chest towards the right leg. Hold the stretch and relax. Repeat with the other leg. If you want to accentuate your hamstrings, then you should perform this stretch with a straight back. If you want to accentuate both the lower back and the hamstrings, then you should round the back more while moving forward towards the knee.

Quadriceps and groin

▼ **Stretch 7:** Lie on your right side with both hips and legs flexed at 90°. Keeping the thighs touching, flex the left knee and grasp the left ankle with the left hand. Exhale and pull the knee back by the ankle so that the left thigh moves into a hyperextended position. Hold the stretch and relax. Repeat with the right leg, lying on your left side.

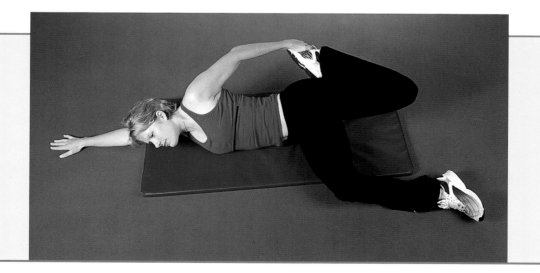

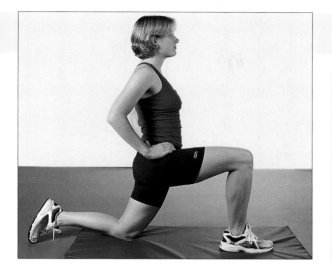

Remember these are general stretches that cover the most important muscle groups. They can be incorporated into any programme as part of a warm-up and cool-down. If you have been pre-scribed another specific stretching routine, then follow that instead.

▲ **Stretch 8:** Place your right leg in front in a lunge posi-tion. Place the left knee on the ground and put your weight on both legs. Maintaining an upright position in the torso and keeping the left knee on the ground, exhale and shift your body weight forward towards the bent right leg. Hold the stretch and relax. Repeat with the other leg.

Hold the stretch and relax. Repeat with the right leg. If this position does not stretch the calf enough, stand fur-ther away from the wall. A variation of this exercise is to bend the back leg and shift your weight backwards, thereby accentuating your Achilles tendon.

Calf muscles

▶ **Stretch 9:** Stand upright facing a wall a short distance away from it and feet together. Step forward towards the wall with the right leg, lean over and, with the palms up against the wall, support your body in a straight-line posi-tion. Keep your left leg extended behind you, the left foot pointing straight ahead and the heel flat on the ground.

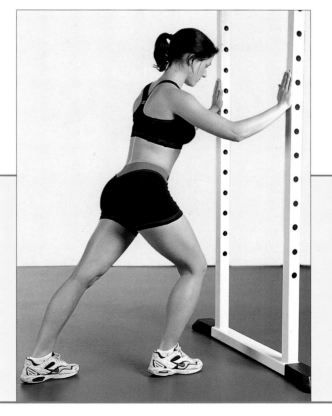

The fundamentals of resistance training

TECHNIQUE

Learn the technique properly. Don't copy other people, for they may be doing it wrong. Your instructor should demonstrate an exercise and then allow you to try it. With more complex exercises, you risk injury if you don't know what you are doing. Always perfect a technique using lighter weights before increasing the load. With technique comes concentration. Before executing a specific exercise, run it through your mind. When performing an exercise, concentrate on the key points provided by your instructor.

BREATHING

In resistance training, you generally always breathe out during an exertion and breathe in during the relaxation phase of a movement. However, many people use a technique called the Valsalva manoeuvre. This involves taking a deep breath and holding it while lifting. It makes you slightly stronger throughout the movement, but it also increases blood pressure drastically, which is not good for your heart and can deprive your brain of oxygen. Besides dizziness and the possibility of fainting, you could burst a blood vessel if the pressure build-up is too high.

Holding your breath increases abdominal pressure during lifting, which increases the compressive force on fluid in the abdominal cavity, thereby providing increased back support and stability. However, the breath does not necessarily have to be held to achieve this effect. By exhaling through pursed lips you can maintain pressure in the abdominal cavity, but prevent it from increasing to the point of becoming a risk.

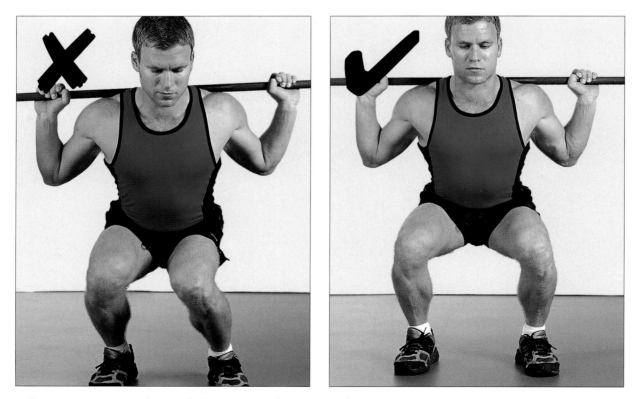

Left: **Incorrect** squatting technique. The knees do not track over the line of the feet (heel-to-toe). Not only can this type of lateral deviation damage the knees and cartilaginous structures, but it is also bad for the lower back and pelvic structures.

Right: The **correct** squatting technique. The body is well balanced and the knees follow the correct movement path.

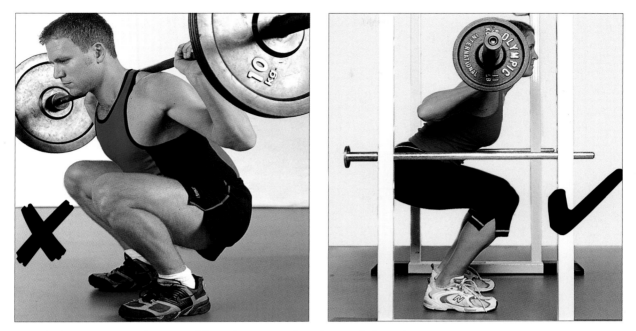

Left: *The deep squat position demonstrated here is* **incorrect** *and can damage the knee joint.*

Right: *In* **correct** *squatting movements the thighs should be parallel to the floor and the knees should not move beyond the toes.*

There is a stage referred to as the sticking point. This is a joint's weakest point in a range of motion and limits how much weight you can lift. When performing an exercise, you can generally feel where your weakest point is. It is standard practice to hold your breath using the Valsalva manoeuvre until you pass this point, after which you begin to exhale through pursed lips.

STABILIZING

Stabilization refers to a condition of being resistant to change. For the weight trainer, it means in practice that a certain part of the body has to resist the forces applied to it when another part of the body is moving. A good example is the bent-over barbell-row. Even though the upper back muscles are used to lift the weights, other muscles have to maintain the bent-over position and supply a resistive force against which the active muscles have to pull. These are called the movement stabilizers. In the case of the bent-over barbell-row, the back extensors, abdominals, gluteus maximus and hamstrings have to act as stabilizers. You have to train these muscles if you want to lift heavier weights.

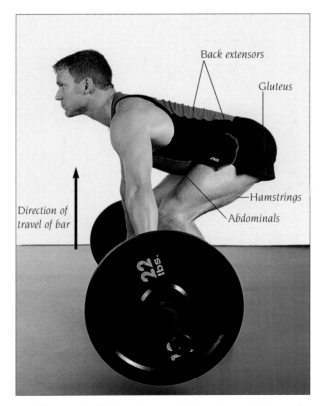

Back extensors

Gluteus

Hamstrings

Abdominals

Direction of travel of bar

In the bent-over barbell-row, the upper back and arm muscles are the primary movers. The lower back, abdominals, buttocks and hamstrings are the stabilizers.

GRIPS

There are various grips in resistance training. Each grip has its own applications. The main grips are as follows:

① The **overhand grip** – palms facing downwards.

② The **underhand (reverse) grip** – palms facing upwards.

③ The **closed grip** – used in most styles. The hands and thumbs wrap around the bar from opposite ends to form a closed circuit. This serves as a safety mechanism, with the thumb acting as a stopper to prevent the bar from slipping out of your hands.

④ The **open grip** – fingers and thumb run in the same direction around the bar in a C-shape, leaving an open end. This is not the norm and can be dangerous when you are lifting heavy weights. Experienced weight trainers use it because it allows for better biomechanical alignment of the joints and because it can reduce loading on the wrist and its soft-tissue structures. However, the bar can slip from your hands and fall with possibly catastrophic consequences.

⑤ The **hooked grip** – a closed-grip variation used in lifts such as the clean-and-jerk, the snatch and deadlifts. The the thumb is wrapped around the bar in a closed grip, but is trapped underneath the fingers. This grip is used when the loads are heavy and when the hand and finger strength might be insufficient to maintain a standard grip on the bar. It helps prevent the bar from slipping from your hands while lifting a heavy weight.

⑥ The **alternated grip** – one hand uses the overhand grip and the other hand the reverse grip. It is mainly used in deadlift variations to avoid all the forces being focused directly on the spine. The alternated grip is stronger and spreads the weight across your spine, with more of the load on the muscles and less on the vertebral column. It does not matter which hand is in the overhand or reverse position, as long as you alternate them between sets. This prevents a side-dominance pattern developing. Spotters (*see p40*) also use this grip to protect their backs.

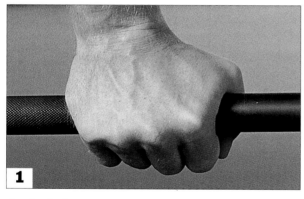

Overhand grip.

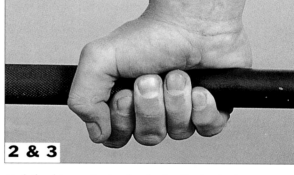

Underhand (reverse) grip, also showing the closed grip.

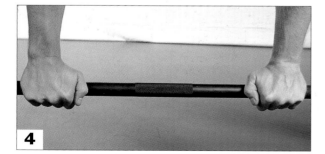

Open grip.

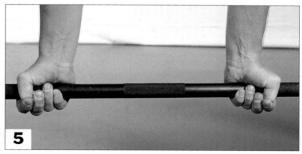

Hooked grip.

⑦ A variation of these grips is the **narrow, wide** and **normal grip length**. The normal grip length is approximately shoulder width apart. The narrow and wide grip lengths are narrower and wider variations of the normal grip, and are used to accentuate different parts of the muscles being trained. Before changing your grip length, consult with your trainer. Irrespective of the length chosen, however, the bar should always be balanced when you lift it.

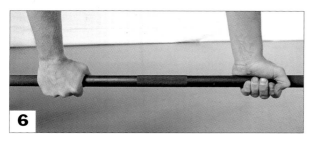

Alternated grip.

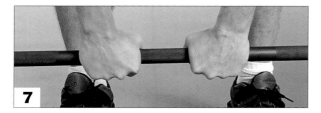

Narrow grip.

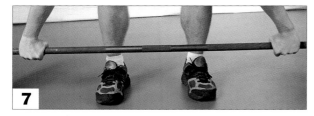

Wide grip.

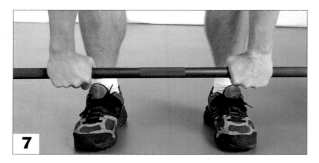

Normal grip.

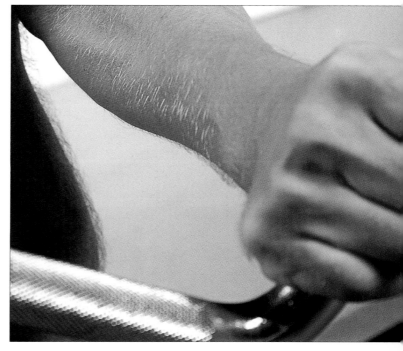

WRIST WRAPS AND GLOVES

Sweat limits your ability to grip a heavy bar. Gym gloves will help. You can also use chalk dust on its own or with wrist wraps. Wrist wraps are often used for Olympic and power lifts due to the heavy weights and particular lifting techniques. They function like the hooked grip, increasing your hold on the bar and providing good wrist support.

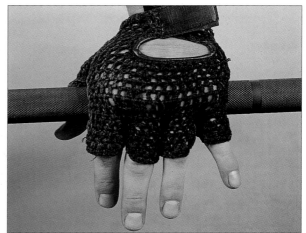

Gym gloves reduce slipperiness due to sweat.

WEIGHT BELTS

Weight belts have unfortunately become a fad in resist-ance training. Olympic and power lifters use them. In exercises that load the spine excessively, they can be used to protect the back when loads approach maximal (90–100% 1RM). One-repetition maximum (1RM) is the maximum weight that you can lift through a complete range of motion, only once, but with good form (*see p*107). A weight belt limits the extent to which the abdominal cavity can expand. This gives the abdominal muscles something against which to contract, thereby increasing fluid pressure in the abdominal cavity. In this way the support-bridge effect on the spine is strengthened.

If you use a weight belt all the time, your body's nat-ural stabilizers are not used to the same extent and therefore are not strengthened as much. As a result, your risk of injury actually increases due to these lesser developed muscles.

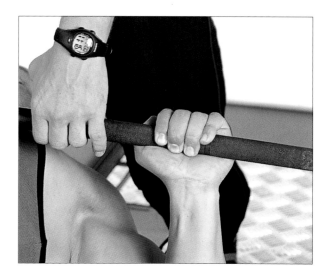

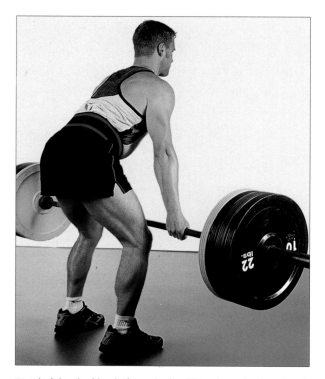

Weight belts should only be used when lifting heavy loads and with exercises that load the spine excessively.

SPOTTING

Spotting is a safety measure when training with heavy weights and in risky exercises. When a person cannot complete the range of motion or would otherwise miss a repetition due to fatigue, a spotter will bear some of the load and assist the lifter to complete the exercise set.

The spotter can help with forced repetitions, a tech-nique used in certain training systems. When the lifter has reached fatigue, and would not be able to lift the weight through another complete repetition unaided, the spotter assists with additional repetitions at the same load.

Most of the time you will not need a spotter, but it is safe practice to use one when performing free-weight exercises that load the back, are above the head and neck, and those that are over the chest. Squats, behind-the-neck presses, bench presses, dumbbell pullovers and pectoral flyes are examples of spotting exercises.

If spotting is done incorrectly, it can injure the spotter or the person lifting the weights. For heavy-weight exer-cises more than one spotter is needed and support must be supplied at both ends of the barbell. For dumbbell exercises, spotters provide support as close to the wrist as possible, and sometimes even on the weights, but not the elbows. Spotters are not used for explosive lifts such as power cleans, clean-and-jerks or snatches, because of the risk of injury to both parties if something goes wrong.

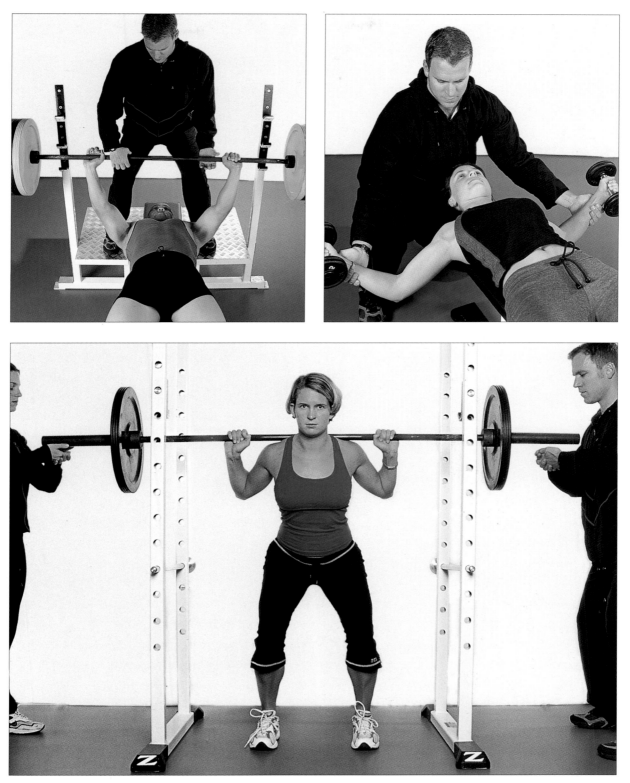

Top left: Spotting technique for the flat bench press. Assist only when the individual achieves muscle failure.

Top right: Dumbbell exercises, like this supine flye, require the spotter to get as close as possible to the weights.

Above: When using heavy weights, as in this back squat, it is prudent to have more than one spotter.

Spotters run the same risk of injury as those performing an exercise, and the same precautions should be taken with regards to technique, preparation and execution. If you are unsure of the correct spotting technique for an exercise, consult your instructor.

PREPARATION

Preparation refers to positioning yourself correctly before lifting weights. This has to do with biomechanics and ensures safety. When lifting a barbell from the ground, you have to position yourself over the bar so that your back is not rounded and you are standing close to it, with the shoulders leading upwards. This will give optimal lifting biomechanics and protect your back. Other considerations are:

- The grip width used (*see p39*).
- The type of grip used (*see p38*).
- Foot positioning.
- The type of breath holding used (*see p36*).
- Head position.
- Back position.

Grip width and the type of grip, and breath holding employed during a lift have already been discussed. The correct **head position** will keep your back slightly arched. You should always look up.

Correct **foot position** will ensure balance and control of the weight during an exercise. Your feet should normally be placed about shoulder width apart with feet slightly turned out. For certain exercises, the feet can be wider, but seldom narrower. A narrow stance will compromise your balance. A strong support base allows you to lift more weights with better balance and coordination. Even with movements such as lunging, the distance between your feet should be maintained for better balance. When lifting barbells, your feet should run underneath the bar with the shins nearly touching it. This improves your line of pull on the bar and shortens the resistance lever so that your back muscles have to work less to lift the bar. Some variations do not fit this rule, but they are exceptions.

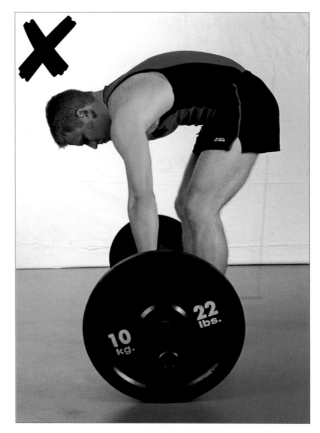

*This shows the **incorrect** way of lifting weights. Bending forward over the barbell like this loads the lower back more than the legs. The lifter runs the risk of injuring his back.*

Another part of preparation is **zipping up**. Before lifting a weight, you should tighten your stomach muscles. This increases stability of the spine (*see p47*).

Keep in mind that your **back** only has a secondary role to play when training (unless you are training the back muscles, of course). Ensure that your posture is such that your back does not bear the load. When lifting a weight from the ground, do not bend forward too much and use your legs to assist you. You should always lead with your head and shoulders.

LOWERING WEIGHTS

Equally important to lifting weights is placing them back on the ground. The key to this is the same as for lifting: keep the bar or dumbbells as close to your body as possible to reduce strain on the back. When returning from a high-

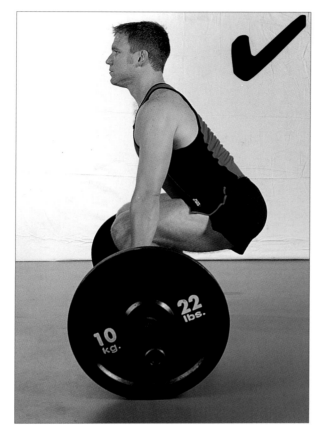

The **correct** lifting position shifts the load to the legs and away from the back. This gives better lifting mechanics and also reduces the risk of injuring the lower back.

lifting position, lower the weight in phases: first allow the arms to straighten, rest them on the legs momentarily, then continue to lower them to the ground by flexing the hips and knees, with straight arms and a slightly arched back.

When lowering weights after seated or supine dumbbell exercises, such as pectoral flyes or dumbbell shoulder presses, lower and bring the dumbbells in towards the stomach, and each other, before trying to get up. Always remember to control the weights on the way down and don't let them fall.

RANGE OF MOTION

Weight training improves flexibility, provided that with each exercise you train through its full range of motion (ROM), from the starting point to the correct finish position. Complete movements actively stretch your muscles and tendons due to the force the weights apply. This not only improves flexibility, as does regular stretching, but also strengthens the muscle along its entire length.

Most exercises are performed using the full range of motion. However, partial repetitions also have value. Should you not be able to complete an exercise's full range of motion due to fatigue, you can perform partial repetitions to fatigue your muscles even more. This is known as the Burn system and is used by many bodybuilders and strength-training athletes. A variation is the supraoverload system, where you train with weights heavier than your one-repetition maximum (100–120% 1RM), but only perform partial repetitions. Both these methods are advanced training systems and should not be tried without a period of preparation, instruction and spotting.

SPEED OF EXECUTION

To avoid using momentum you should take 1–2 seconds to lift a weight; and to limit the risk of injury 2–4 seconds to lower it. However, this can be adapted to achieve different training goals.

What you need for effective resistance training

Effective training requires medical clearance, good technique and form, and the discipline to persevere over time.

MEDICAL CLEARANCE

Have a medical check-up before you start resistance training. Your current health status will guide the fitness professional in establishing a suitable training programme for you.

Anyone can benefit from resistance training, but certain conditions may require you to train under medical supervision. Examples are: osteoporosis, osteoarthritis, fibromyalgia, cardiovascular disease, coronary artery disease, diabetes (Type I and II), chronic obesity, chronic pulmonary disorders such as asthma and cystic fibrosis, any recent surgical procedure, or pregnancy.

TECHNIQUE AND POSTURE

Poor technique and form limits your progress and increases your risk of injury.

DISCIPLINE

Resistance training is taxing on your body and can create a significant amount of discomfort during its initial phases. It takes discipline to work through the discomfort, not pain, and to carry on. You will feel a difference after two to three weeks, but visible results require at least four to six weeks of regular training. Even though you do not see much change initially, the long-term health benefits are nevertheless substantial.

Safety in the weight room

Your safety depends on how careful you are and on your consideration for others. Your personal trainer and the gym management should inform you about the risks of training and about the gym's safety procedures. Safety should be considered when: adding and removing weights; spotting; moving around the weight room; and storing equipment.

ADDING AND REMOVING WEIGHTS

When adding or removing weights to a suspended barbell, remember that the bar is always loaded on both sides. If someone adds or removes all the weights from

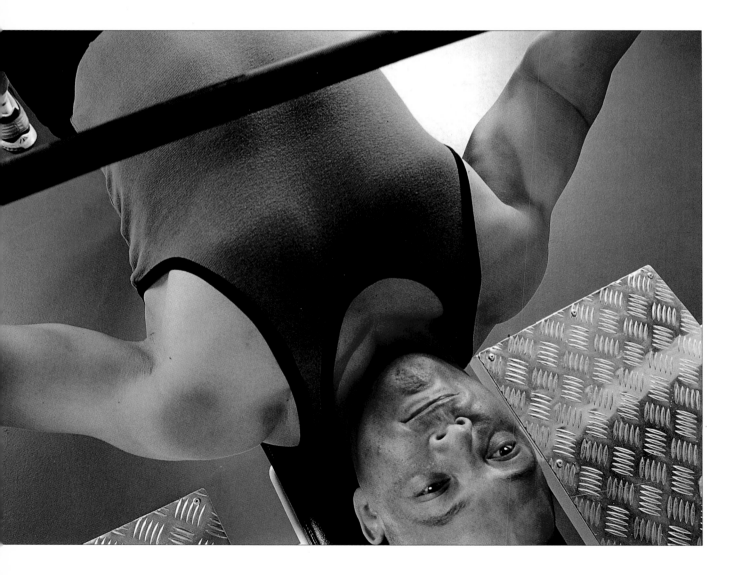

one side, the bar could suddenly swing upward and cause injury. Instead, ascertain the weight of the bar and the weights to be added or removed and then load or unload the bar gradually and evenly on both sides.

Exercise machines should also be loaded and unloaded with care. A common apparatus that causes injury is the squat/calf-raise machine. Some individuals are too lazy to climb underneath the machine to squat upwards to the starting position. Instead, they lift the shoulder pads and use the pull-pin to keep the shoulder pads suspended. When they're done, they leave the pull-pin inside the weight stack without resetting the shoulder pads. The next person, wanting to add or remove weights from the bar, may pull the pin while standing under the shoulder pads. This will cause the shoulder supports to fall on the base of the person's neck or head, which can result in a broken neck and even paralysis.

When working with barbells and dumbbells, always check and tighten the locks against the weights before performing an exercise.

SPOTTING

If you are training with heavy weights and are unsure of yourself, ask someone to assist or spot. You also need a spotter when you are pushing your limit. The spotter only assists when you cannot lift the weights to completion, or if, for example, you are performing a heavy bench press and failure would result in injury. With the aid of a spotter, you can safely push yourself further and therefore develop faster. Ask someone training with you or ask an instructor to spot for you.

MOVING AROUND THE WEIGHT ROOM

Pay attention to what is happening around you, especially in the free-weight area of the gym. If you don't watch where you are going, you could walk into a barbell being lifted, resulting in injury to the lifter as well as yourself. If the person loses control of the barbell, other people in the vicinity could also be injured. Most injuries of this kind occur during overhead barbell and dumbbell exercises and those with significant lateral movement such as pectoral flyes. Try not to move backwards in the training area, and always take note of who is doing what before moving.

EQUIPMENT STORAGE

When dumbbells and barbells are left lying about, people can trip over them. If you are carrying weights, this can be catastrophic. Return the weights to their place when you are finished with them. Also remember to leave bars on their supports where applicable, such as in the case of bench presses.

Basic safety concerns

Training should be fun and enjoyable and should not involve unnecessary risk. There are rules that can ensure safe training.

WARM-UP SETS

Whether you have just been introduced to resistance training or are participating in an advanced training programme, always add one or two warm-up sets (groups of repetitions) to every exercise to prepare the muscles. The loads used for the warm-up sets should be lighter than the minimum load for the day. For example, if you are training using four sets with weights at 70% of your one-repetition maximum you can introduce two warm-up sets: one at 50% and the other at 60% of 1RM. This progressively activates the muscles and reduces the risk of injury.

TECHNIQUE, TECHNIQUE, TECHNIQUE

When learning a new exercise, use a light load. Continue with this load until your instructor is satisfied that your technique has been perfected before progressing to heavier weights. This also applies when you have not trained for a while: start with light loads and only progress once your exercise technique is back on par with what it used to be. Do not try any exercise without proper instruction by a qualified instructor. Deviation from the correct technique could lead to abnormal forces being applied on your joints, joint capsules, muscles and tendons, and this can result in injury.

BOUNCING

When performing exercises, you shouldn't bounce at the bottom of the movement because high eccentric forces can cause muscles and cartilage to tear. When performing resistive plyometrics, for example, in the jump squat, where the bar is placed on the shoulders, this is standard procedure, but athletes using this technique are usually trained and conditioned for this. The average gym member is not conditioned to tolerate these forces and is therefore susceptible to injury.

NO PAIN, NO PAIN

Forget no pain, no gain; the real saying is, no pain, no pain. It is as simple as that. If something hurts, don't do it. Reduce the weights if you are feeling pain. If the pain disappears, you can carry on, but if it persists you should stop and seek medical advice from someone specializing in exercise therapy.

PROTECT THE KNEES

You can reduce the risk of injury to your knees by training with good form and technique. Loads and repetitions should be increased gradually in consultation with a fitness professional.

In any squatting or lunging movement, the knee should pass over the line of the foot, namely from heel to toe, and preferably not past the toes. If it deviates laterally from this path, too much rotational force is applied to the knee joint, which can cause an injury.

Another cause of injury is the depth of the squat and the degree to which the knee is bent as a result. The correct technique for a squat is to bend your knees only until

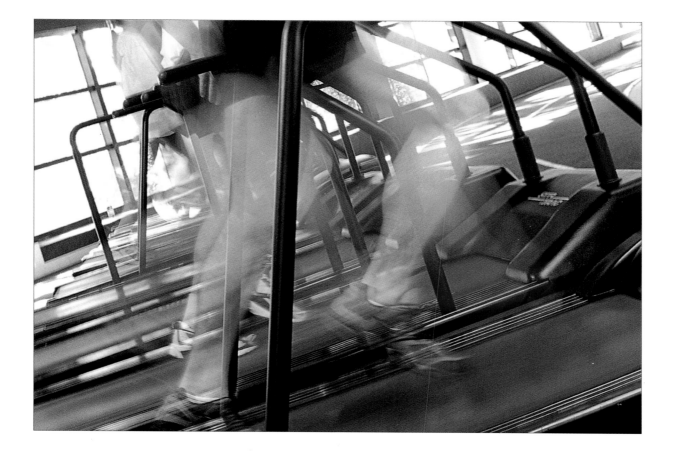

your thighs are parallel to the floor. Ask a fitness professional to evaluate and correct your technique if necessary. You can also monitor your form by watching yourself in a mirror.

PROTECT YOUR BACK

Many exercises focusing on a total-body workout involve the lower back musculature to a large extent, either in stabilization or in a functional role.

Protecting the lower back does not mean wearing a weight belt for every exercise. You should instead be using and training your back's natural stabilizers, such as the abdominals and vertebral extensors. Contracting the deep abdominal muscles and slightly arching the lower back will protect the intervertebral disks against unnatural compressive forces and injury. Tightening the abdominals before lifting is also known as zipping up.

The abdominal cavity primarily consists of internal organs and fluid. Fluids are incompressible. By contracting the abdominal muscles during an exercise, this fluid-filled compartment forms a support bridge for the vertebral column as it is placed under pressure by muscle contraction. It is assumed that this fluid pressure, induced by contraction, assists in supporting the weights and thereby reduces the load on the back extensors.

Etiquette

Every gym has written and unwritten rules.

EQUIPMENT SET-UP

When you have added weights according to your prescribed training programme, replace them on the weight racks when you are finished.

When finished on a machine, remove the weight-stack pin and place it on the lowest weight setting and reset the other components, such as the shoulder pads, that could possibly injure someone. When using dumbbells, return them to their weight racks when finished. Do not leave them lying around.

SEVEN PRINCIPLES OF RESISTANCE TRAINING

Individuality: Each person responds differently to a programme.

Motivation and drive: To get optimal results from resistance training, you must be able to push yourself to failure in an exercise, work through muscle soreness and stick it out.

Nutrition: To replace the energy and repair the muscles you have used during training, you need to increase your intake of carbohydrates and, to a lesser extent, protein. Consult a dietician.

Progressive overload: Your workload needs to be increased (gradually) on a regular basis for your muscles to keep developing.

Regularity of training: Train at least two to three times a week to see reasonable results, but three to five times a week is recommended.

Rest: It is during the rest period that your body regenerates, adapts and becomes stronger.

Safety: Safety first and results second.

HAND TOWEL

Place a hand towel on the machine while exercising and towel off the seat or bench afterwards. Nobody wants to use a machine when the seat or bench is dripping with someone else's sweat. If you do not train on a towel, at least wipe the seat or bench afterwards. This also helps extend the functional life span of equipment.

TIME ON EQUIPMENT

Restrict your time on the equipment, especially if people are waiting to use it after you. Offer to share it if you see someone queuing up. While you are resting between sets, the other person can perform exercises and vice versa. This is common practice among regular gym members and need not distract you from training effectively.

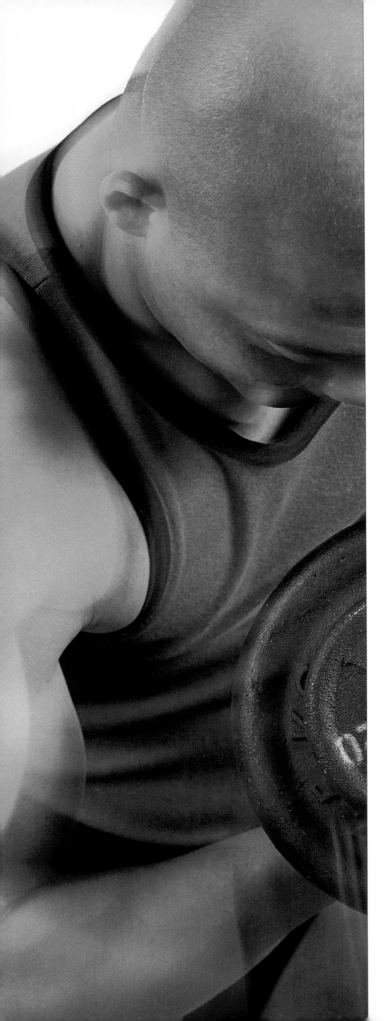

Resistance-training exercises

Besides having the correct exercise technique, you need a programme with a selection of exercises, with recommended loads and numbers of repetitions structured according to your current status and with your training goals in mind.

The four categories of exercises are: core exercises; structural exercises; power exercises and auxiliary exercises.

Core exercises

Core exercises such as bench presses are complex multijoint exercises incorporating primary movements around major joints and they involve large muscle groups.

Structural exercises

Structural exercises such as squats are variants of core exercises, where the spine is loaded and the back stabilizes and sometimes assists the movement.

Power exercises

Power exercises, such as snatches, are explosive structural exercises.

Auxiliary exercises

Auxiliary exercises are mainly single-joint movements such as dumbbell lateral raises. However, some multijoint movements such as lat pulldowns, that do not conform to core exercise criteria, are also described as auxiliary.

An exercise session should start with core, structural

Cautionary note: Women are generally asked to direct the bar or weight in the chest exercises to approximately 2cm above the base of the breastbone or sternum. In the case of men, it will be the nipple line. Instructions to lift a load to the upper or lower chest are directed at both men and women.
All reference to 'arching' the back refer to making the back hollow, as opposed to rounded.

or power exercises, before the muscles are fatigued, so that good form can be maintained. One should not do more than two to four of these in one session.

Resistance-training programmes should aim at training all the main muscle groups equally. The same applies to more advanced forms, such as split programmes, except that in that case exercises are split over different days with more allocated per body part.

When developing programmes for specific sports (a subject not covered in this book), the procedure becomes complex as it requires analysis of movement patterns, seasonal fluctuations and energy-system training.

This section will show examples of exercises for the different parts of the body with numerous exercises allocated to each muscle group.
Each exercise will be described under the following headings: • classification • primary muscles targeted • starting position • execution.
Variations of the exercises are mentioned only to serve as a starting point for research into additional weight-training practices and exercises.
! This icon indicates that the exercise should not be attempted without prior instruction from a qualified professional. Incorrect execution could lead to injury.

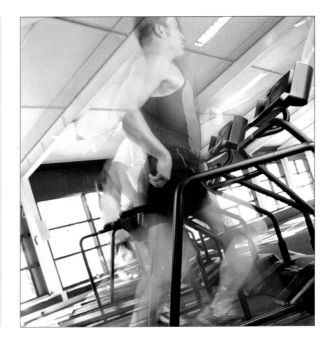

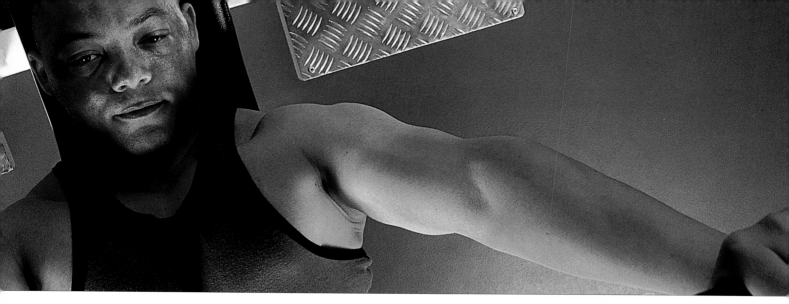

Chest

▼ Straight-arm pullover (dumbbells)

Classification: Auxiliary. **Primary muscles:** Pectoralis, latissimus dorsi (lower) and serratus anterior muscles.

Starting position: Feet are placed on the floor slightly wider than shoulder width apart. Rest the dumbbell upright on the bench between the legs, while still in a seated position. Grasp the dumbbell under its top weight plate. When lying back on the bench, bring the dumbbell to the chest. Extend the arms and push the dumbbell upwards over the chest.

Execution: Keeping the elbows slightly flexed throughout, lower the dumbbell in an arced motion behind the head until it is just below the shoulder line. Keep the hips against the bench. Push the dumbbell back to the starting position.

Variation: Execute with bent arms, or use a barbell instead of dumbbells.

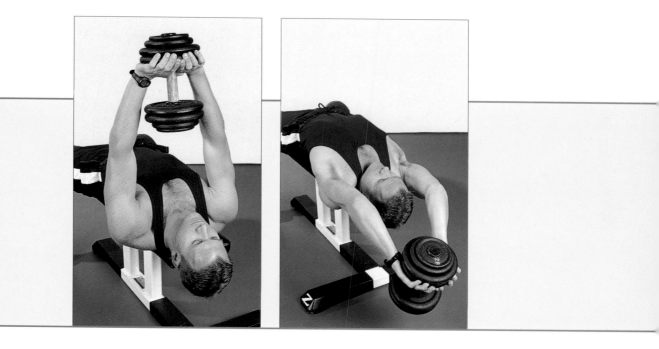

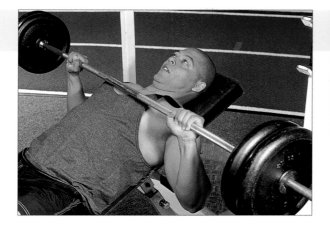
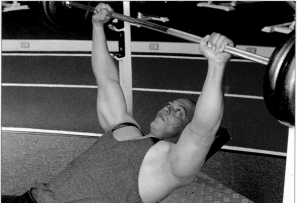

! ▲ Incline bench press (barbell)

Classification: Core. **Primary muscles:** Pectoralis major (upper), anterior deltoid, triceps.

Starting position: Lie back on the incline bench with your feet shoulder width apart on the floor. Using an overhand closed grip, with hands 7–10cm (3–4in) wider than shoulder width apart, lift the bar off its supports and extend your arms above the upper chest and shoulders.

Execution: Lower the bar towards your nipple line slowly until it touches your chest. Push the bar up in an arced motion until your arms are extended above your shoulders. If you lower the bar to a higher position on the chest, you accentuate the anterior deltoid muscles rather than the pectoralis muscles.

Variation: Execute with narrower and wider grips, Smith Machine or dumbbells.

▼ Machine flye (Pec-deck)

Classification: Auxiliary. **Primary muscles:** Pectoralis major (middle), anterior deltoid.

Starting position: Adjust the height of the machine seat, if necessary. Push your forearms against the pads and form a 90° angle between elbow and shoulder joint.

Execution: By controlling the elbows backwards, stretch the chest and shoulders wide open and then contract these muscles and push the pads inwards as far as possible. Hold this position briefly and control back to the starting position.

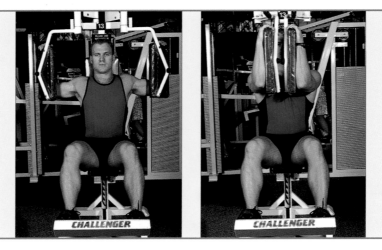

▶ Flat bench press (dumbbells)

Classification: Core. **Primary muscles:** Pectoralis major (middle), anterior deltoid, triceps.

Starting position: Rest the dumbbells on the knees while in a seated position. Use an overhand closed grip with your palms facing each other. Lie back on the bench and bring the weights to the sides of the chest. Feet are placed either on the floor shoulder width apart, on the bench or lifted in the air. Extend the arms and push the dumbbells up above the chest until they touch each other. Turn the hands inwards, so that the palms are facing the front.

Execution: Slowly lower the dumbbells towards the nipple line and the sides of the chest (do not go below the line of the chest) and then push upwards until you are back in the starting position.

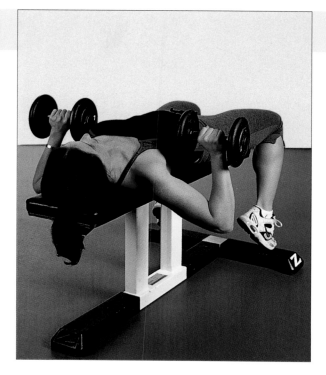

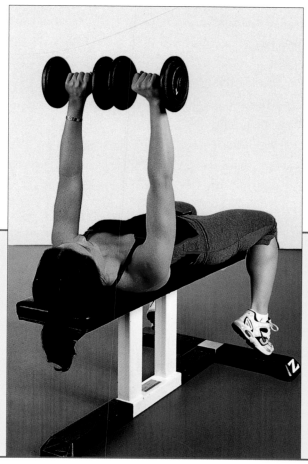

▶ Supine flye (dumbbells)

Classification: Auxiliary. **Primary muscles:** Pectoralis major (middle), anterior deltoid.

Starting position: Rest the dumbbells on the knees while still in a seated position. Use an overhand closed grip with palms facing each other. Lie back on the bench and bring the weights to the sides of your chest. Feet are placed either on the floor shoulder width apart, on the bench or lifted in the air. Extend the arms and push the dumbbells up over the chest until they touch each other.

Execution: Flex the elbows slightly and maintain this position throughout. Control the weights sideways away from the body until the arms are open wide on either side and the chest is expanded. Do not allow the dumbbells to go beyond the depth of your shoulders. Using the same arced motion, push the weights back to their starting position.

Variation: Incline flye.

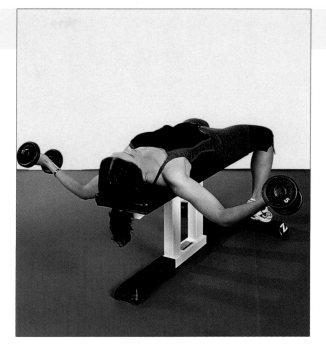

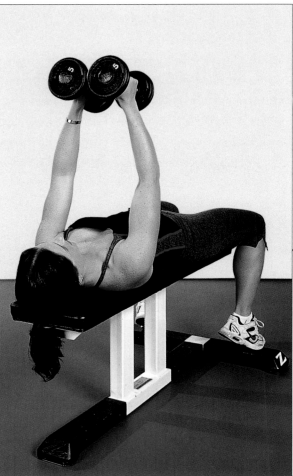

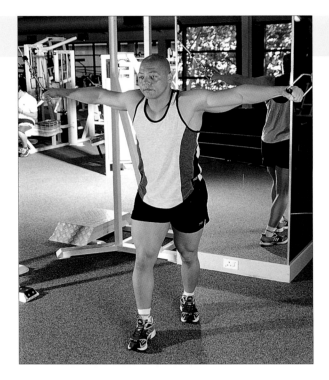 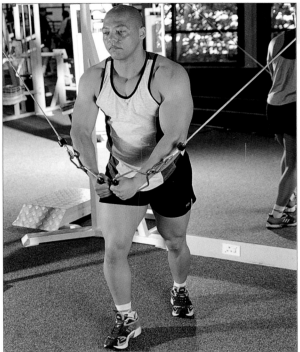

▲ Cable crossover

Classification: Auxiliary. **Primary muscles:** Pectoralis major (middle and lower), anterior deltoid.

Starting position: Hold each handle of the pulley machine with an overhand grip, your palms facing down. Keeping your arms up at shoulder height with the elbows slightly bent, step forward with one leg until you are supporting the weights. Stand with one foot in front and one foot behind for better support. Keeping the back straight, lean slightly forward.

Execution: Open the arms and expand the chest slightly without discomfort. Pull the cables forward and downward in an arcing motion until the hands meet in front of the navel. Hold briefly and resist the cables eccentrically back to the starting position.

Variation: Execute with single arms.

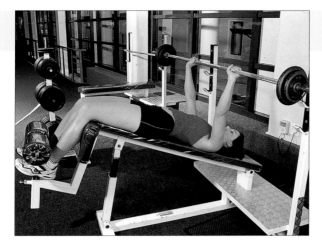 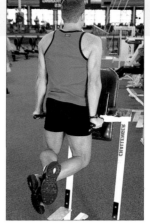 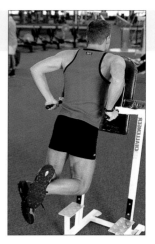

! ⬍ Decline bench press (barbell)

Classification: Core. **Primary muscles:** Pectoralis major (lower), anterior deltoid, triceps.

Starting position: Use an overhand closed grip with your hands 7–10cm (3–4in) wider than shoulder width apart. Secure your ankles and feet in the shin pads provided. Lift the bar off the supports and extend the arms upwards.

Execution: Slowly lower the bar towards the nipple line until it touches the chest, and then slowly push it upwards in an arced motion until the arms are extended above the shoulders.

Variations: Execute with narrower and wider grips, Smith Machine or dumbbells.

▲ Dip

Classification: Auxiliary. **Primary muscles:** Pectoralis major, pectoralis minor, anterior deltoids, triceps.

Starting position: Keeping the knees flexed, support the body on extended arms.

Execution: Lower your body by flexing your elbows until they are just below 90°, or as far as possible within comfort, and allow them to move slightly outwards. Slowly push the body upwards back to the starting position.

Variation: Execute with weights around your ankles; dip machine.

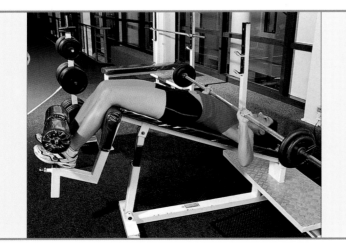

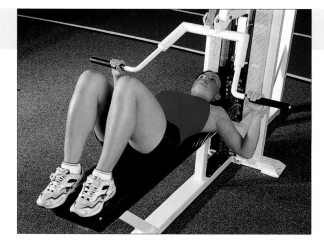

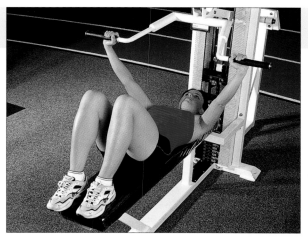

▲ Bench-press machine

Classification: Auxiliary. **Primary muscles:** Pectoralis major (middle), anterior deltoid, triceps.

Starting position: Use an overhand closed grip with hands 7–10cm (3–4in) wider than shoulder width apart. When lying down, the handgrips should be in line with the nipple line. Feet are placed on the floor slightly wider than shoulder width apart, on the bench, or lifted in the air.

Execution: Lift the machine bar and extend the arms upwards. Slowly lower the grips until they are as close to the chest as possible. Push the bar upwards until the arms are extended.

▼ Machine chest press

Classification: Auxiliary. **Primary muscles:** Pectoralis major (middle), anterior deltoid, triceps.

Starting position: Sit on the chest-press machine with your back right against the support. Make sure its handles are aligned with your nipple line. Adjust the seat if necessary. Take hold of the handles with an overhand closed grip.

Execution: Push and extend the arms forwards. Hold briefly and control back to the starting position.

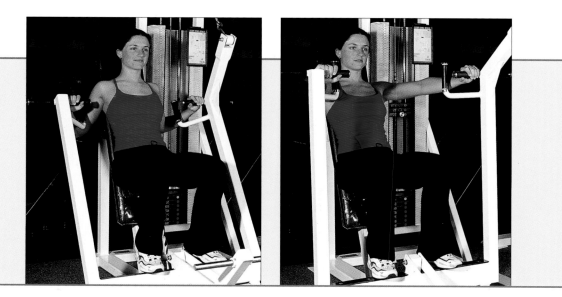

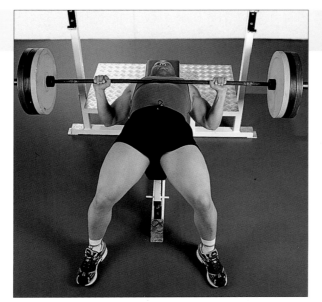
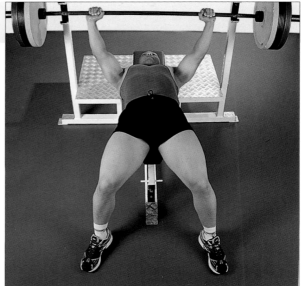

! ▲ Flat bench press (barbell)

Classification: Core. **Primary muscles:** Pectoralis major (middle), anterior deltoid, triceps.

Starting position: Use an overhand closed grip with your hands 7–10cm (3–4in) wider than shoulder width apart. This exercise will be executed in the same way as for decline barbell bench presses, except that the bench used is flat, and there are no shin pads. Your feet should be placed either on the floor shoulder width apart, on the bench or lifted in the air. Your back will be better protected should your feet be on the bench or lifted, but you are limited in this position as to the load you can lift due to balance. So, to lift more weight, keep your feet either on the ground or on a platform. Lift the bar off its supports and extend the arms upwards.

Execution: Lower the bar towards your nipple line slowly until it touches your chest. Push the bar up in an arced motion until the arms are extended above the shoulders.

Variation: Execute with narrower and wider grips or with the Smith Machine.

Upper back and shoulders

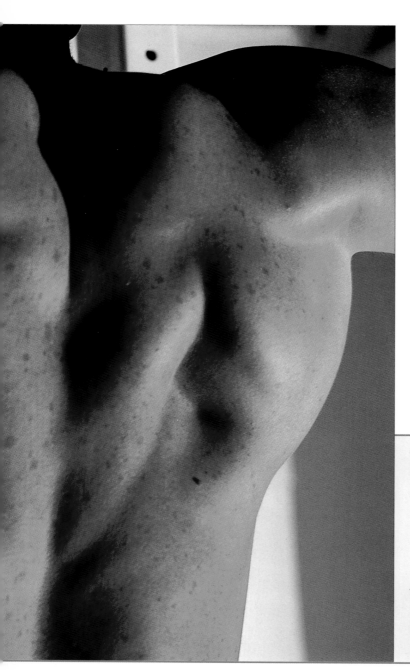

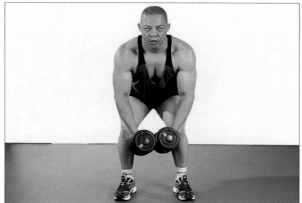

▲ Reverse flye (dumbbells)

Classification: Auxiliary. **Primary muscles:** Deltoids (posterior and middle), trapezius (upper), rhomboids.

Starting position: Hold the dumbbells with an overhand grip, palms facing each other. Stand with your upper back straight, knees slightly bent. Your feet should be shoulder width apart. Bend forwards in the hips until your torso is just above parallel to the ground and your lower back is slightly arched. Extend your arms downwards, but keep the elbows slightly flexed throughout.

Execution: Maintaining your elbow position, lift the weights laterally in an arced motion until your arms are parallel to the ground. Hold briefly and return to the starting position.

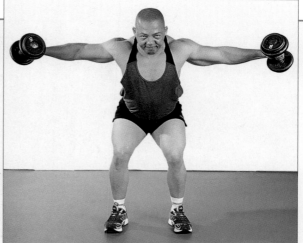

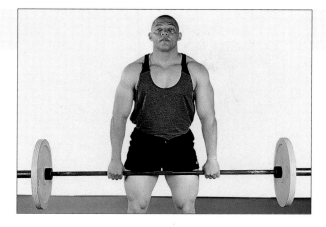

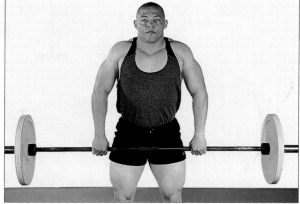

▲ Shoulder shrug (barbell)

Classification: Auxiliary. **Primary muscles:** Trapezius, rhomboids.

Starting position: Grasp the barbell with an overhand grip and your hands shoulder width apart. Stand up, keeping your knees slightly bent and your feet also shoulder width apart. Bend your elbows slightly and rest the bar on your thighs.

Execution: Raise the barbell by lifting your shoulders towards your ears without using your arms. Hold briefly, and lower the barbell as far down as you can, without losing form, and repeat.

Variations: Lift and roll backwards; lift and roll forwards; execute with dumbbells hanging at your sides.

▼ Upright row

Classification: Auxiliary. **Primary muscles:** Trapezius, anterior deltoid.

Starting position: Stand upright. Hold the bar with an overhand grip, with hands about 10cm (4in) apart. Keep it hanging at arm's length.

Execution: Leading with your elbows high, lift the bar until it reaches your upper chest. Hold briefly and return to the starting position.

Variation: Execute with narrower and wider grips or with dumbbells.

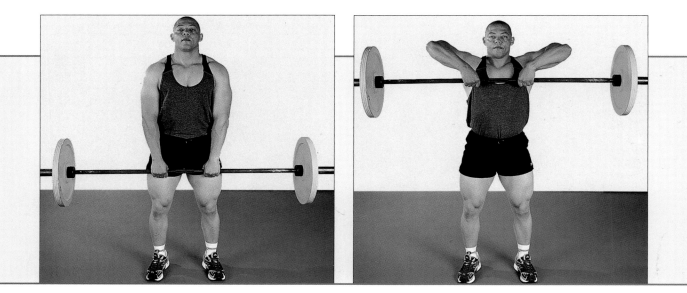

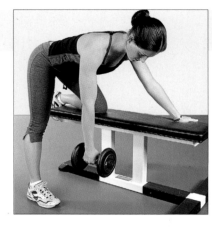
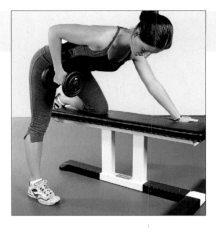

▲ Bent-over dumbbell-row

Classification: Auxiliary. **Primary muscles:** Latissimus dorsi, trapezius, biceps.

Starting position: Support your body on your left knee and extended left arm on the flat bench. Take the dumbbell in the right hand with an overhand grip, palm facing the body. Slightly arch the lower back and bend forward until your torso is parallel to the ground and your right arm is extended downwards.

Execution: Keeping the right elbow tight against the body, pull the dumbbell straight up, with the elbow leading, until you touch your ribs. Hold briefly and control back to the starting position. Alternate each set.

▼ Machine shoulder press

Classification: Auxiliary. **Primary muscles:** Deltoid (anterior and middle), trapezius (upper), triceps.

Starting position: Sit on the machine. Adjust the seat so that when you grasp the handles there already is tension in your shoulder muscles. Hold the handles using an overhand grip with your hands 7–10cm (3–4in) wider than shoulder width apart.

Execution: Push the handles upwards until your arms are extended overhead. Hold briefly and return to the starting position.

Variation: Execute with narrower and wider grips, and with different shoulder press machines.

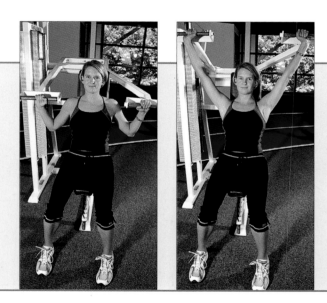

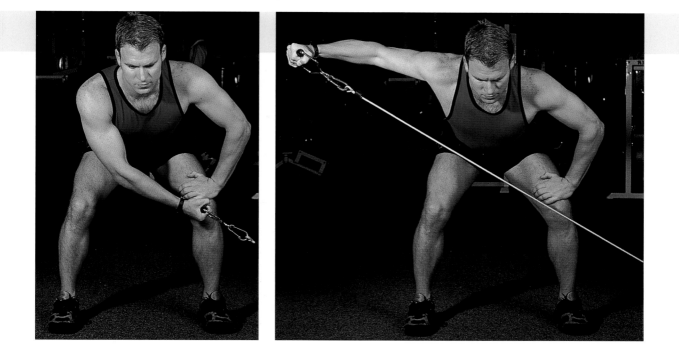

▲ Bent-over cable-lateral

Classification: Auxiliary. **Primary muscles:** Deltoids (posterior and middle), trapezius (upper), rhomboids.

Starting position: Stand sideways between the pulleys with your back straight and your knees slightly bent. Your feet should be shoulder width apart. Bend forwards in the hips until your torso is parallel to the ground and your lower back is slightly arched. Support your left arm on the left thigh and grasp the bottom left handle of the pulley with the right hand. Keep your elbow slightly flexed throughout.

Execution: Maintaining your elbow position, pull the cable laterally upwards in an arced motion until your arm is parallel to the ground. Hold briefly and return to the starting position. Alternate each set.

Variations: Bent-over cable-lateral crossover; single reverse flye (dumbbells).

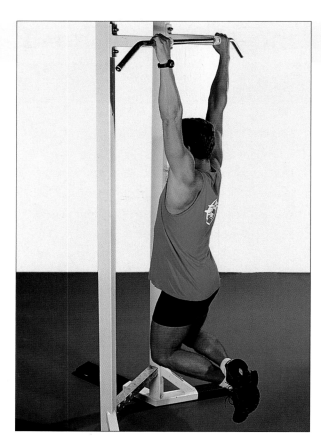

◄ Chin-up

Classification: Auxiliary. **Primary muscles:** Latissimus dorsi, trapezius (upper), biceps, brachialis.

Starting position: Grasp the chin-up bar with an overhand grip and your hands shoulder width apart. Hang with your arms extended and your knees flexed.

Execution: Pull your body up vertically until your chin passes the bar. Hold briefly and control your movement back until your arms are extended.

Variations: Execute with narrower and wider grips; reverse-grip chin-up; behind-the-neck chin-up; weighted chin-up.

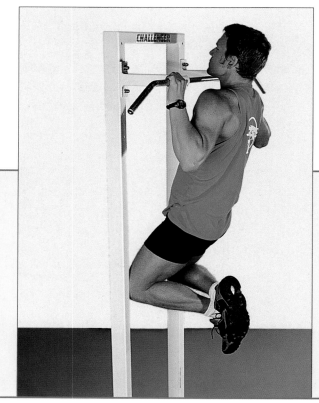

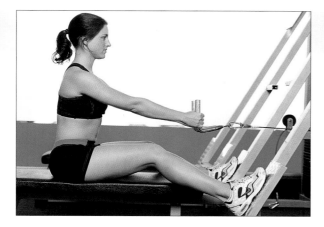 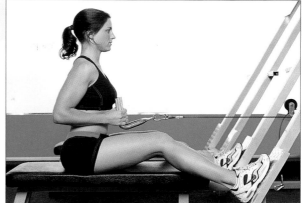

▲ Seated cable/pulley row

Classification: Auxiliary. **Primary muscles:** Trapezius (middle), latissimus dorsi, rhomboids.

Starting position: Sit with your feet braced against the footplate. Bend the knees and bend forwards in the hips, taking hold of the handles. Straighten the legs, but keep the knees slightly bent. Maintain a normal arched lower back position. Extend the arms in front of you and stretch the upper back.

Execution: Maintain the slight forward lean during the exercise, but do not move back and forth in the hips. With the elbows moving back past the sides, pull the bar towards the lower chest until it touches. At the same time pull the shoulder blades towards each other. Hold briefly and return to the starting position.

Variation: High-pulley row.

▼ Rowing torso machine

Classification: Auxiliary. **Primary muscles:** Deltoids (posterior), rhomboids, trapezius.

Starting position: Sit with your arms crossed and between the pads of the machine. Ensure the pads are at shoulder height by adjusting the seat.

Execution: Stretch your upper arms forwards as far as you can. Then push the pads with your elbows as far back as possible. Hold briefly and return to the starting position.

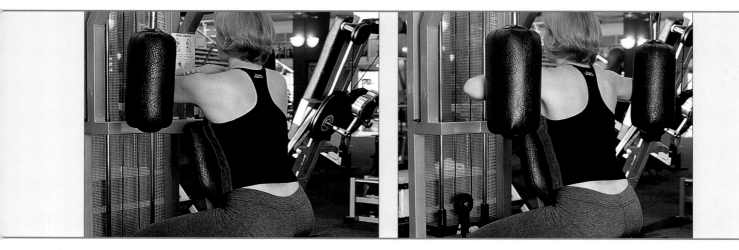

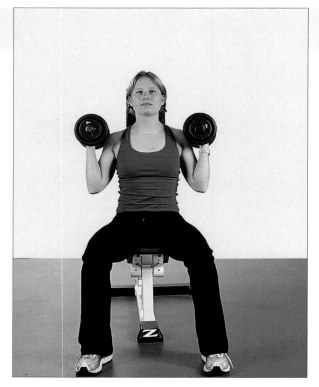 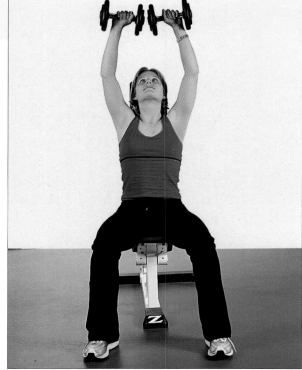

▲ Dumbbell overhead press

Classification: Core. **Primary muscles:** Deltoid (anterior and middle), trapezius (upper), triceps.

Starting position: Sit on the vertical bench with your feet shoulder width apart. Grasp the dumbbells with your palms facing each other. Lift the dumbbells to shoulder height as you sit back.

Execution: Extend your arms and push the dumbbells upwards. While the dumbbells are moving up, rotate both hands so that the palms are facing towards the front of the body when your arms are extended overhead. Hold briefly and return to the starting position.

Variations: Seated front dumbbell press (with palms facing front of the body throughout); Arnold press (start with palms facing chest).

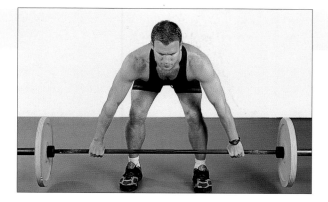
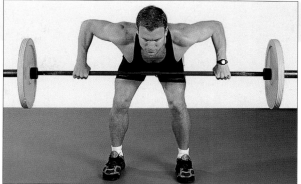

! ▲ Bent-over barbell-row

Classification: Auxiliary. **Primary muscles:** Latissimus dorsi, trapezius, biceps.

Starting position: Stand with your feet shoulder width apart. Take hold of the barbell with an overhand grip with hands also about 10–15cm (4–6in) wider than shoulder width apart. Lift the bar and stand up. Once balanced, slightly arch your lower back, bend the knees and bend forwards in the hips until your torso is parallel to the ground and your arms are extended. Remember to keep your knees slightly bent at all times.

Execution: Pulling up with your upper back and arms, elbows leading, lift the bar towards your lower chest. Limit the upward movement of the torso to about 5cm (2in). Hold briefly and control the bar back to the starting position.

Variation: Execute with T-bar or long-bar rows.

▼ Lat pulldown

Classification: Auxiliary. **Primary muscles:** Latissimus dorsi, posterior deltoids, trapezius (upper), biceps.

Starting position: Facing the lat pulldown machine, take hold of the bar in a wide overhand grip. Sit down and fix your lower legs and thighs under the pad supports. Lean back slightly, with your arms extended overhead.

Execution: Pull the bar downwards and in front of you until the bar touches your upper chest. Hold briefly and control the movement back to the starting position.

Variations: Behind-the-neck pulldowns, alternated front and back.

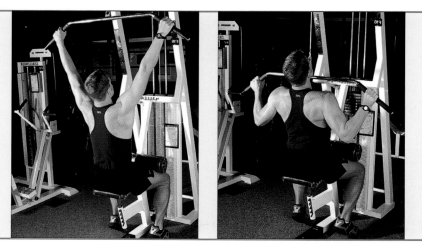

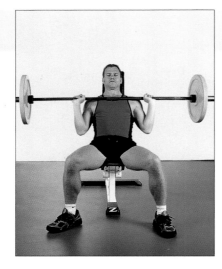
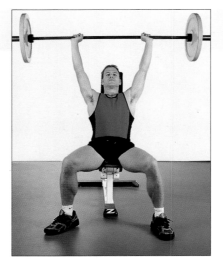

▲ Military press

Classification: Core. **Primary muscles:** Deltoid (anterior), triceps.

Starting position: Sit on the vertical bench with your feet shoulder width apart. Grasp the bar in an overhand grip with your hands 7–10cm (3–4in) wider than shoulder width apart. Extend the bar above your head and shoulders.

Execution: Lower the bar in front of your head until it reaches the front of your shoulders. Push it back up to the starting position.

Variation: Execute with narrower and wider grips.

! ▼ Behind-the-neck press

Classification: Core. **Primary muscles:** Deltoids (posterior), trapezius (upper), triceps.

Starting position: Sit on the vertical bench with your feet shoulder width apart. Grasp the bar in an overhand grip with your hands 7–10cm (3–4in) wider than shoulder width apart. Extend the bar above your head and shoulders.

Execution: Lower the bar behind your head just below ear level. Push it back up to the starting position.

Variation: Execute with wider grip; alternate back and front.

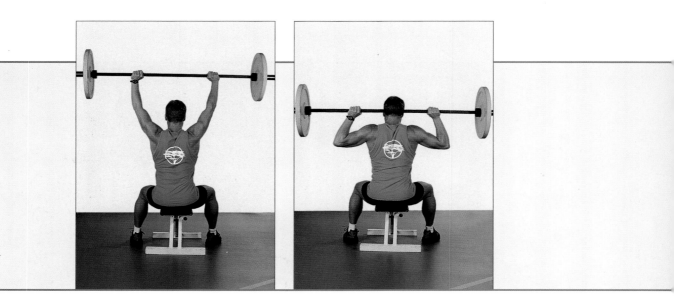

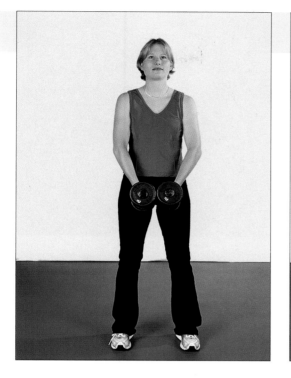
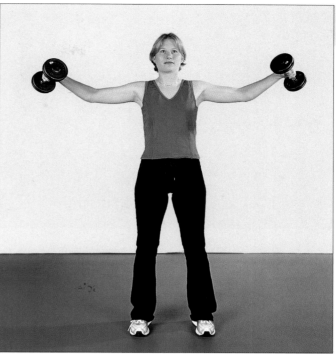

▲ Lateral dumbbell raise

Classification: Auxiliary. **Primary muscles:** Deltoids (middle), trapezius (upper), supraspinatus.

Starting position: Stand with your back straight, knees slightly bent and the dumbbells resting on your thighs. Your feet should be shoulder width apart. Grasp the dumbbells with your palms facing each other. Keep the elbows slightly flexed throughout.

Execution: Maintaining this position, lift the dumbbells laterally upwards in an arced motion until the upper arms are parallel to the ground. Hold briefly and return to the starting position.

Variations: Externally rotate the shoulder (not from the wrist) by turning the thumbs upwards while lifting the dumbbells; front dumbbell-raise; cable side-lateral; cable front-raise; cable lateral-crossover; high-pulley variations

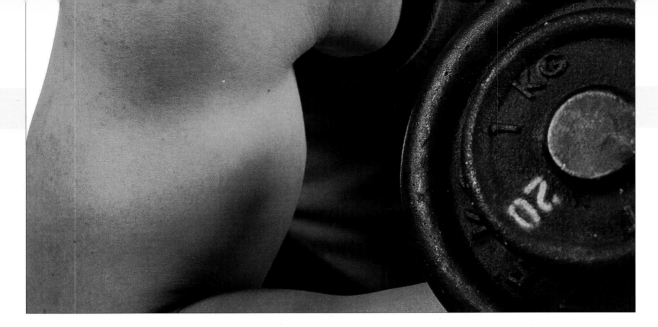

Upper arms

▼ Standing barbell curl

Classification: Auxiliary. **Primary muscles:** Biceps brachii, brachialis.

Starting position: Stand with your feet shoulder width apart and your back straight. Grasp the bar with a reverse grip, hands shoulder width apart, and extend your arms. Rest the bar on your thighs.

Execution: Flex your elbows to curl the bar up towards your chest. Hold briefly and control the movement back to the starting position.

Variations: Reverse barbell curl (using an overhand grip and concentrating more on the brachialis and brachio-radialis muscles – usually performed with a cambered or EZ-bar); standing cable curl.

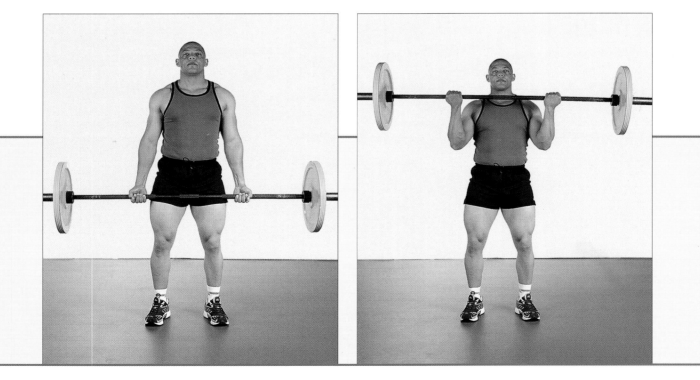

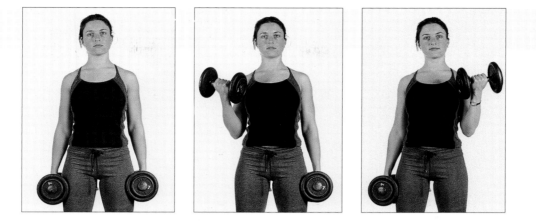

▲ Alternated dumbbell curl

Classification: Auxiliary. **Primary muscles:** Biceps brachii, brachialis.

Starting position: Stand with your feet shoulder width apart and your back straight. Grasp the dumbbells with palms facing each other and extend your arms with the dumbbells hanging at your sides.

Execution: Flex your elbow to curl the right dumbbell upwards towards your shoulder and externally rotating your wrist so that your palm is facing you on completion of the movement. Hold this position briefly and control your arm back to its starting position. Repeat on the left side and alternate.

Variation: Hammer curl (with thumbs facing up, palms facing each other and no rotation).

▼ French press (overhead press)

Classification: Auxiliary. **Primary muscles:** Triceps brachii.

Starting position: Sit on the flat bench with feet about shoulder width apart. Take hold of the dumbbell with its top plates supported in both hands and the thumbs wrapped around the bar. Sitting upright with a slight forward lean, lift the dumbbell upwards, extending the arms so that it is overhead.

Execution: Without allowing the upper arms to move, control the dumbbell downwards behind the head by flexing the elbows until your forearms and biceps touch each other. Push the dumbbell back to the overhead starting position.

Variation: Standing; execute with EZ-bar; overhead-pulley tricep extension.

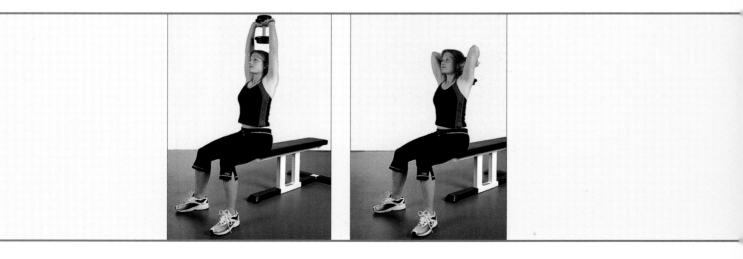

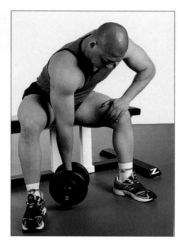
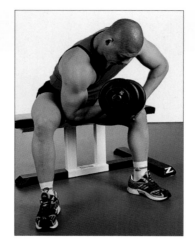

▲ Concentration curl

Classification: Auxiliary. **Primary muscles:** Biceps brachii, brachialis.

Starting position: Sit on a flat bench with your legs wider than shoulder width apart. With the right hand, grasp the dumbbell in a reverse grip. Supporting yourself with your left arm on your left thigh, bend forwards in the torso and hang your right arm between your legs. Do not support it against the inner thigh; let it hang freely. You should not use your inner thigh to assist.

Execution: Flex your elbow to curl the dumbbell up towards your shoulder. Hold briefly and control back to its starting position.

Variation: Cable concentration curl.

▼ Preacher curl

Classification: Auxiliary. **Primary muscles:** Biceps brachii, brachialis.

Starting position: Sit on the preacher curl bench and grasp the bar (preferably an EZ-bar) with a reverse grip, your hands shoulder width apart. Extend your arms down against the bench and keep your upper arms there at all times.

Execution: Flex your elbows to curl the bar upwards towards the chest. Hold briefly and control back to its starting position.

Variation: Machine curl.

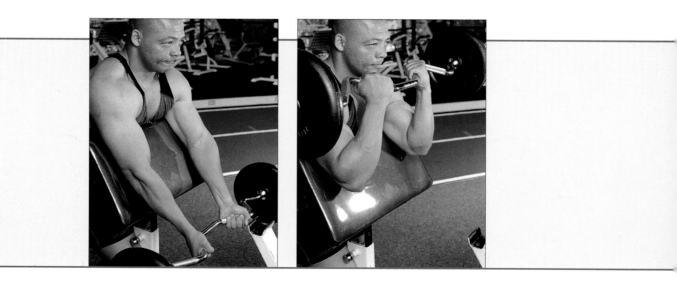

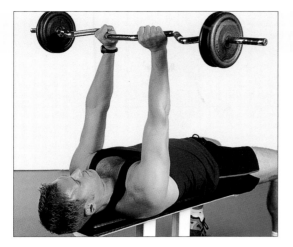

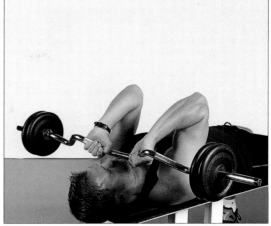

! ▲ Supine tricep press (Skull crusher)

Classification: Auxiliary. **Primary muscles:** Triceps brachii.

Starting position: Grasp the bar (preferably an EZ-bar) with an overhand grip, your hands shoulder width apart. Lie supine on a flat bench with feet straddled on either side of it. Push the barbell upwards, extending the arms above the chest.

Execution: Keeping the elbows pointing up and the upper arms fixed, lower the bar towards your forehead by flexing the elbows. Just before the barbell touches your forehead, push it up to its starting position.

▼ Narrow-grip bench press

Classification: Auxiliary. **Primary muscles:** Triceps brachii, deltoids (anterior), pectoralis.

Starting position: Grasp the bar with an overhand grip, your hands approximately 10cm (4in) apart. Lie supine on a flat bench with feet straddled on either side of the bench. Push the barbell upwards, extending the arms above the chest.

Execution: Lower the barbell towards the centre of the chest. Just before it touches the chest, push it upwards to the starting position.

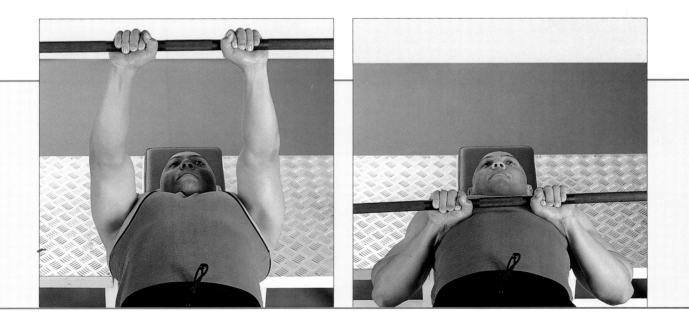

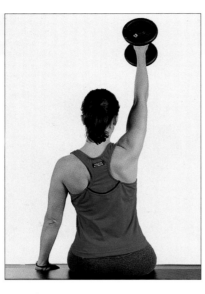
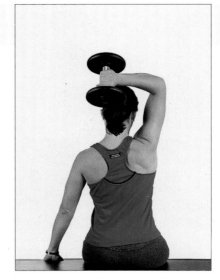

▲ One-arm dumbbell press

Classification: Auxiliary. **Primary muscles:** Triceps brachii.

Starting position: Sit on a flat bench with your left arm stabilizing your body. Hold a dumbbell with the right hand using an overhand grip. Lift the dumbbell, extending the arm overhead.

Execution: Lower the dumbbell behind the head until your forearm is parallel to the ground. Hold briefly and push back to the extended overhead position.

▼ Dumbbell kickback

Classification: Auxiliary. **Primary muscles:** Triceps brachii.

Starting position: Grasp the dumbbell with your right hand, palm facing your body. Support your body on your left knee and extended left arm on the flat bench. Tuck your right arm tight against the side of your body, flexed at the elbow, the upper arm parallel to the ground.

Execution: Maintaining the upper arm position, slowly extend the forearm and hold briefly. Lower the dumbbell slowly to the starting position.

Variation: Cable tricep kickbacks.

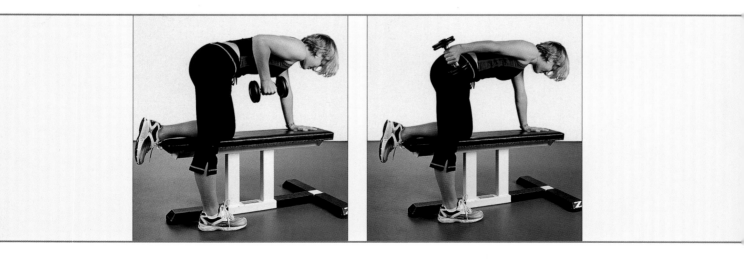

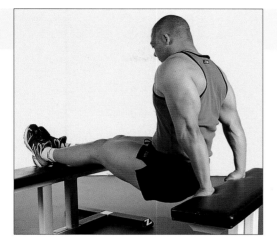
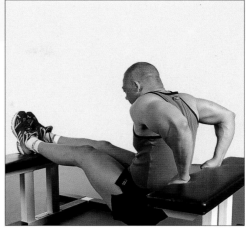

▲ Bench dip

Classification: Auxiliary. **Primary muscles:** Triceps brachii.

Starting position: Place two flat benches about 1m (3ft) apart and parallel to each other. Support your upper body on the bench behind you with your hands shoulder width apart and your arms extended. Place your heels on the bench in front of you and keep your legs straight.

Execution: Lower the body by slowly bending the arms until they go beyond 90°. Slowly push back up to the starting position by extending your arms.

Variation: Place a weight on top of your thighs.

▼ Tricep pressdown

Classification: Auxiliary. **Primary muscles:** Triceps brachii.

Starting position: Using either an angled or a T-bar on the high pulley, grasp the bar with an overhand grip. Stand with your legs shoulder width apart and knees slightly bent. Pull the bar down until your elbows are flexed and pushed against the sides of your body.

Execution: Moving only the forearms, extend your arms downwards. Hold briefly and control back to the starting position.

Variation: Execute with a reverse grip.

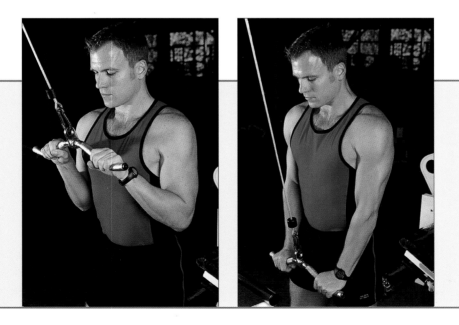

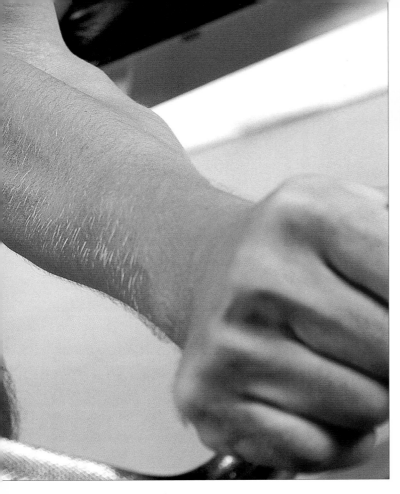

Forearms and wrists

▼ Barbell wrist curl

Classification: Auxiliary. **Primary muscles:** Wrist flexors.

Starting position: Grasp the barbell with a reverse grip and sit on a flat bench. Rest your forearms on your thighs, with the barbell hanging over the knees. Lean slightly forwards in the torso. Open your hands and lower the bar by rolling it to your fingers.

Execution: Raise the bar up by curling the fingers and the wrists as much as possible. Hold briefly and control the movement back to the starting position.

Variations: Execute with dumbbells or with cables; reverse barbell wrist curl; ulna and radial deviation.

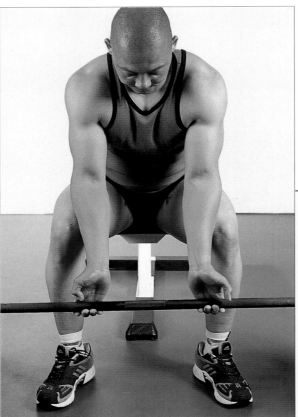

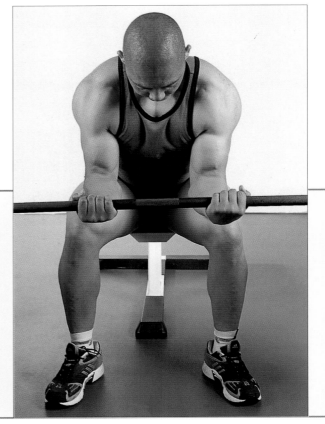

Lower back

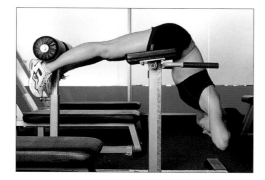 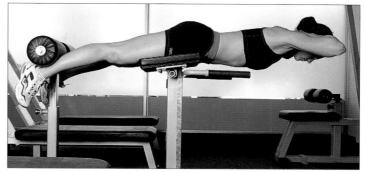

! ▲ Prone back-extension

Classification: Auxiliary. **Primary muscles:** Erector spinae, gluteus maximus.

Starting position: Lock legs under the support pads and lie prone over the Roman bench with your hips hanging over the edge. Lower your torso by bending in the hips so that your head and upper body are hanging down. Place your hands behind your neck.

Execution: Raise your torso upwards until it is just about parallel to the ground. Hold briefly and control the movement back down to the starting position.

Variations: Execute with weights or with rotations, to the left and to the right; glut-ham gastroc raise.

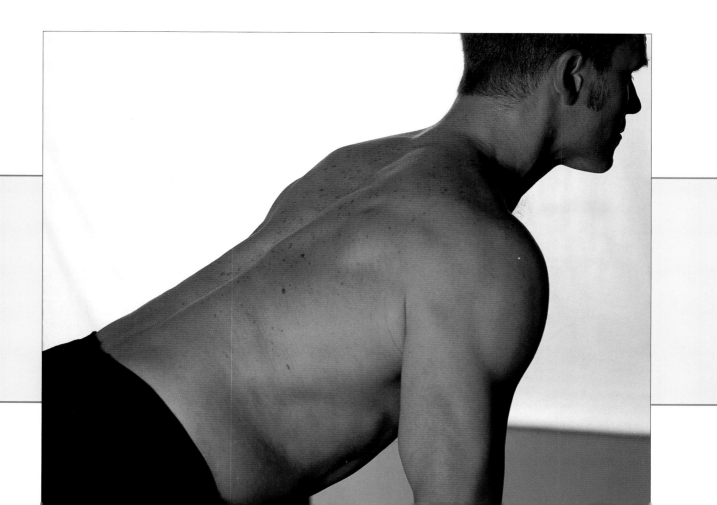

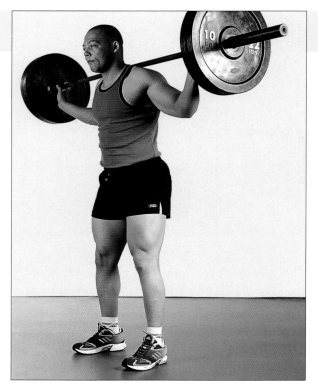
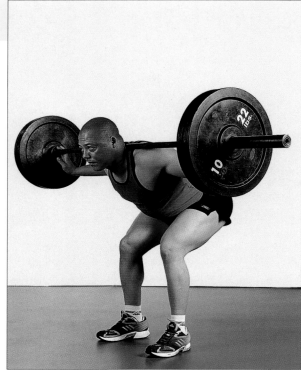

! ▲ Good morning (bent leg)

Classification: Structural. **Primary muscles:** Gluteus maximus, hamstrings, erector spinae, abdominals.

Starting position: Grasp the bar with an overhand grip. Stand upright with the bar supported at the base of your neck and your feet also shoulder width apart. Keep your lower back slightly arched, and your head up.

Execution: Bend forwards in the hips and knees until your torso is parallel with the ground. Maintain an arched lower back throughout. Hold briefly and stand up again into the starting position.

Variation: Stiff-legged good morning accentuates the hamstrings.

! ▼ Deadlift (bent leg)

Classification: Structural. **Primary muscles:** Gluteus maximus, hamstrings, erector spinae.

Starting position: Stand in front of the barbell with your feet shoulder width apart. Bend down using your hips and knees and grasp the bar with an alternated, hooked grip, using the outside of the knees as an indicator of where to hold. Maintain a slightly arched lower back, knees bent and head up.

Execution: Using the lower back, hips and thighs, stand up with your arms extended. Lead with the head and shoulders. When the bar passes the knees, push the hips forwards, shoulders back and chest out, until the bar is resting against the thighs and you are standing upright. Hold briefly and control the bar back down to the starting position. Alternate your hand position between sets.

Variations: Stiff-leg deadlift accentuates hamstrings; Romanian deadlift; rounded-back deadlift (performed on a bench using the stiff-leg position, but rounding the back while lowering the weights, and using only the erector spinae muscles to lift the weights. Do not use this variation without proper conditioning and instruction).

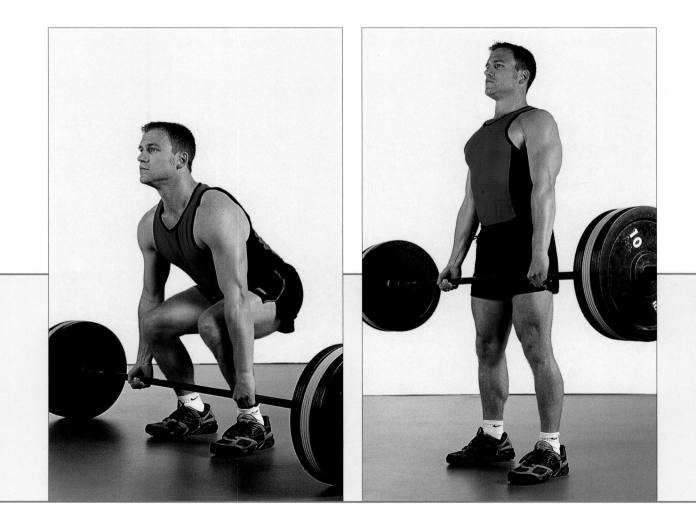

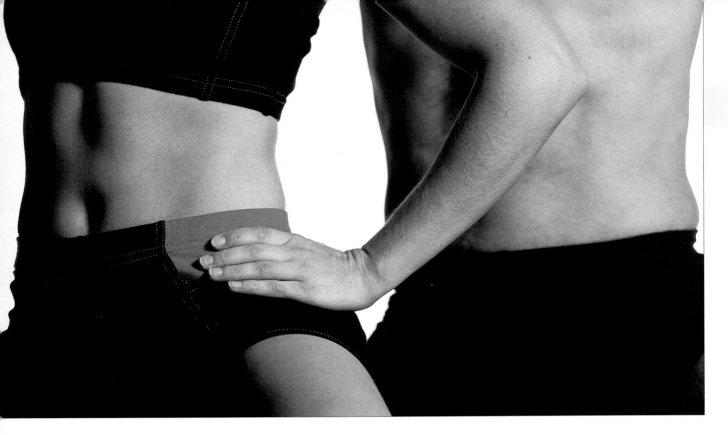

Abdominals and torso

▼ Crunch

Classification: Auxiliary. **Primary muscles:** Rectus abdominus (upper).

Starting position: Lie supine with bent knees and your back flat on a mat or abdominal bench. Place your hands behind your neck.

Execution: Use your upper torso at all times without lifting your lower back off the ground. Curl the shoulders and upper back in and upwards, lifting them off the floor with elbows moving towards the thighs. Hold briefly and lower yourself back to the starting position. To increase the intensity of this exercise, keep your head and neck off the ground, thereby maintaining tension in the abdominals, or increase the angle of the bench.

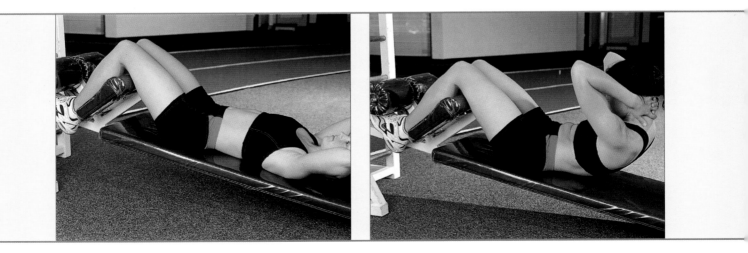

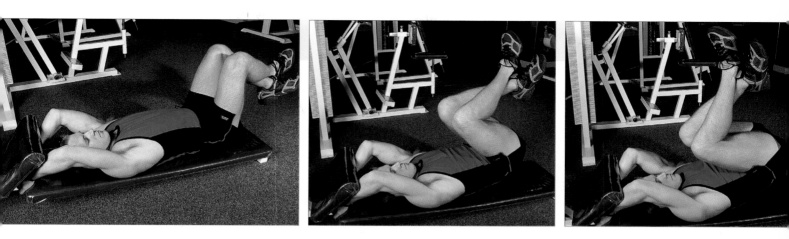

▲ Reverse crunch

Classification: Auxiliary. **Primary muscles:** Rectus abdominus (lower).

Starting position: Lie supine with your knees bent and back level on a mat or flat bench. Stabilize your body by holding on to something immovable behind your head. Lift your feet and keep your hips and knees flexed.

Execution: Curl your knees towards your chest until your lower back has lifted off the ground. Now that your lower back is lifted, contract your abdominal muscles even more and lift your hips higher. Hold briefly, then control back to the starting position. Keep your upper body still throughout.

Variation: Straight legs.

▼ Twist crunch

Classification: Auxiliary. **Primary muscles:** Rectus abdominus (upper), serratus anterior, obliques.

Starting position: Use either a mat or an abdominal bench. Lie supine with knees bent and back flat on the ground. Place your left hand behind your neck. Lift your right foot and rest it on the left knee. Stabilize the right side by extending the right arm laterally on the floor.

Execution: Use the upper torso at all times without lifting the lower back off the ground. Curl the left shoulder and upper back upwards towards the right knee, lifting them off the floor. Hold briefly and lower back to the starting position. Alternate sides after each set. To increase the intensity of this exercise, keep your head and neck off the ground, thereby maintaining tension in the abdominals.

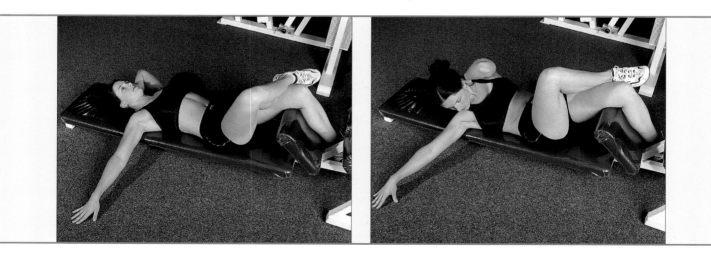

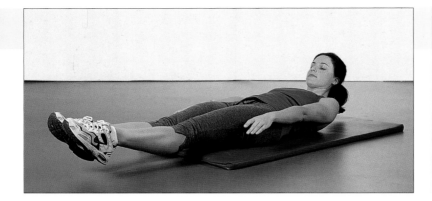

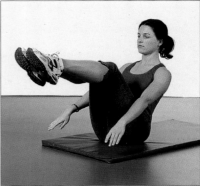

▲ Knee-tuck

Classification: Auxiliary. **Primary muscles:** Rectus abdominus (lower), hip flexors.

Starting position: Lie supine with your legs extended, arms against your sides and your back as flat as possible on the ground. Lift your head and curl your upper back and shoulders off the ground.

Execution: Simultaneously raise your upper torso and pull your knees in towards your chest. Keeping your head up at all times, slide your hands forwards past your legs as you do so. Hold briefly and control back to the starting position until your legs are extended a little above the ground. Keep your upper back slightly raised off the ground.

Variations: Knee-up, where the hands support the upper body at a 45° angle from behind and the knees are tucked into the chest; V-up.

▼ Machine crunch

Classification: Auxiliary. **Primary muscles:** Rectus abdominus (middle and lower).

Starting position: Sit with your back against the support and hold the handles. Secure your feet against the footplate. Hold the top pad against your upper back throughout.

Execution: Pull your body as far forwards and downwards as the machine will allow. Hold briefly and control to the starting position.

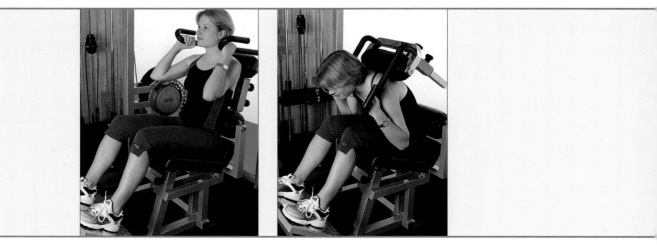

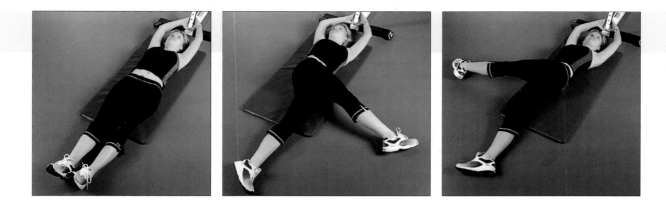

! ▲ Lying crossover

Classification: Auxiliary. **Primary muscles:** Obliques and hips.

Starting position: Lie supine and hold on to something immovable just behind your head. Extend your legs and keep them flat on the ground.

Execution: Keeping your shoulders and upper back against the ground, lift your right leg and swing it over the left leg so that it is as close to the left shoulder as possible. Return to the starting position and alternate legs.

▼ Hanging leg raise

Classification: Auxiliary. **Primary muscles:** Rectus abdominus (lower), serratus anterior, hip flexors.

Starting position: Support your body weight on the horizontal arms. Hang your legs down so that your body is vertical. Bend your knees slightly and maintain this angle throughout.

Execution: Raise your legs slowly to hip level. Hold briefly and control back to the starting position. Do not swing.

Variation: Bent-leg knee raise.

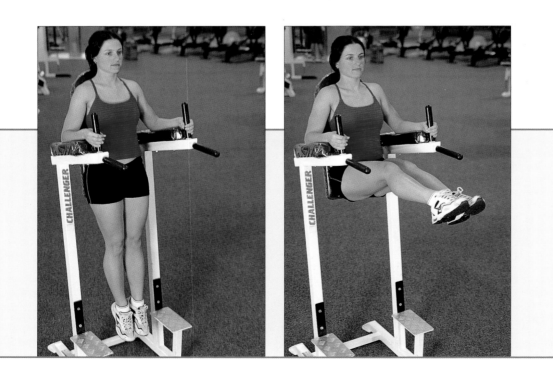

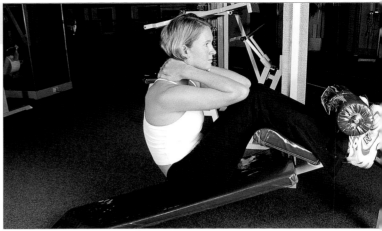

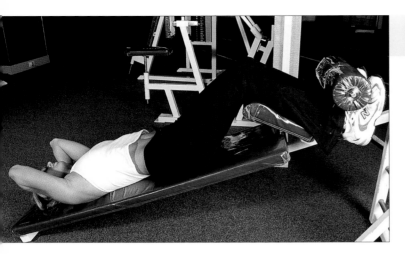

▲ Incline sit-up

Classification: Auxiliary. **Primary muscles:** Rectus abdominus (upper), hip flexors.

Starting position: Hook your feet in the incline-bench footpads and keep your knees bent at approximately 45°. Place your hands behind your neck.

Execution: Curl your neck towards your chest and lift your torso upwards until your elbows touch your knees. Hold briefly and lower yourself back to the starting position.

Variation: Execute with a twist or change the bench angle.

▼ Side raise

Classification: Auxiliary. **Primary muscles:** Obliques, serratus anterior, intercostals.

Starting position: Lie on your right side with your left leg crossed over your right leg, which should be slightly behind the line of your body. Support your body with your right arm by extending it and placing your right hand as close to your right hip as you can.

Execution: Raise your body upwards and away from the right supporting arm by lifting your upper hip as high as you can. Hold briefly and control back to the starting position. Alternate each set.

Variations: Dumbbell side-bend; cable side-bend; with weights.

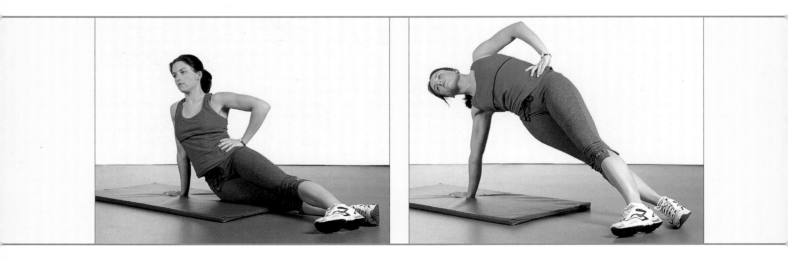

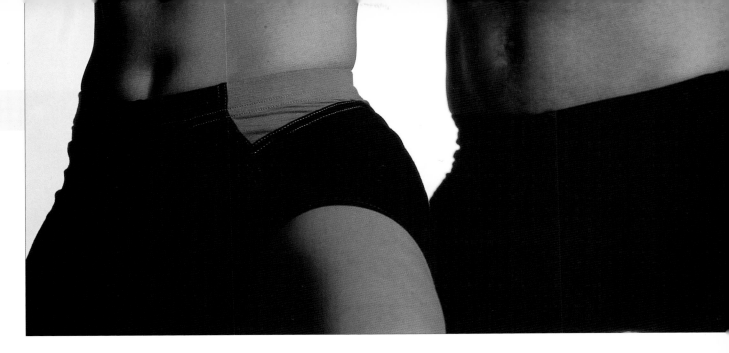

Hips

▼ Cable leg-lift

Classification: Auxiliary. **Primary muscles:** Hip flexors (iliopsoas, rectus femoris, sartorius) and rectus abdominus.

Starting position: Stand with your back to the pulley with its strap on your right ankle. Stand away from the pulley to tension the cable and extend the leg backwards. Hold on to something such as a bench or support bar.

Execution: Lift the back leg upwards and forwards as far away from the pulley as is possible. Hold briefly and control your leg back to the starting position. Alternate legs after each set.

Variations: Execute with hands on hips for balance; cable knee-lift.

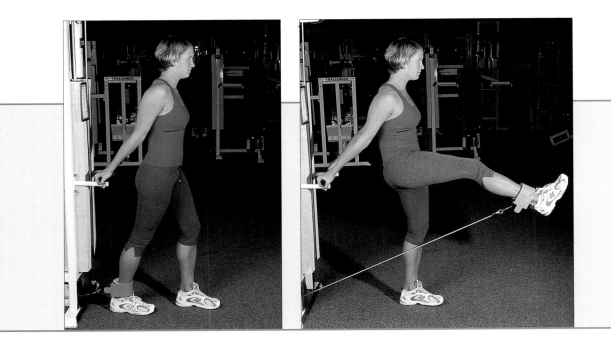

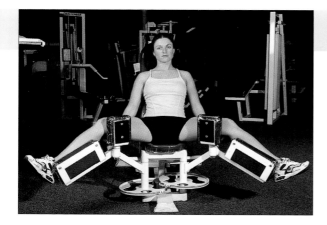

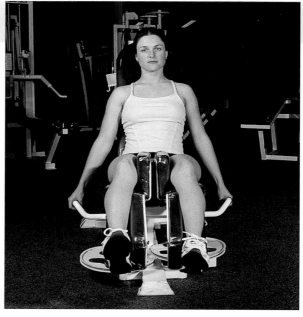

▼ Hip-abductor machine

Classification: Auxiliary. **Primary muscles:** Hip abductors (gluteus medius, gluteus minimus, tensor fascia latae).

Starting position: Sit against the back support of the hip-abductor machine with your legs extended straight in front of you between the pads. Grab hold of the handles on the sides.

Execution: Push your legs as wide open as possible. Hold briefly and return to the starting position.

Variations: Seated and standing cable hip-abduction; total hip machine.

▲ Hip-adductor machine

Classification: Auxiliary. **Primary muscles:** Hip adductors.

Starting position: Sit against the back support of the hip-adductor machine with your legs spread open outside the pads. Grab hold of the handles on the sides of the hip-adductor machine.

Execution: Pull your legs together. Hold briefly and return to the starting position.

Variations: Seated and standing cable hip-adduction; total hip machine.

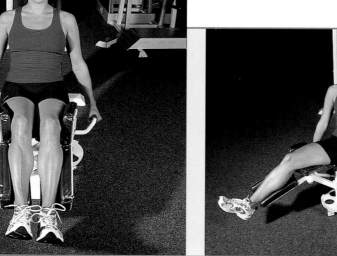

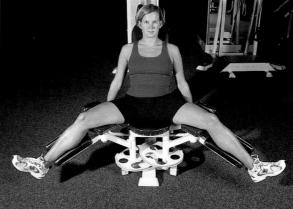

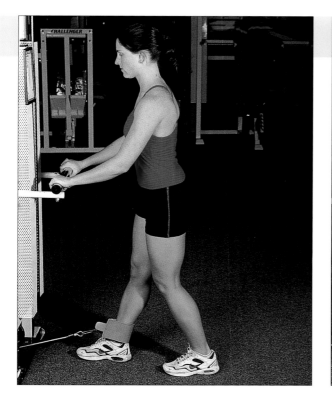
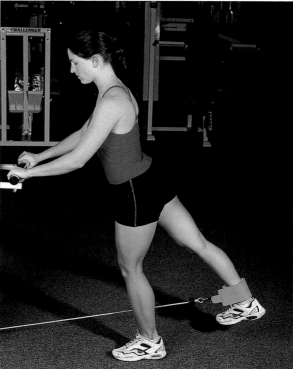

! ▲ Cable kickbacks

Classification: Auxiliary. **Primary muscles:** Hip extensors (gluteus maximus, biceps femoris).

Starting position: Stand facing the pulley with its ankle strap on your right ankle. Stand away from the pulley to tension the cable and pull the leg forwards. Hold on to something such as a bench or support bar.

Execution: Pull your straight leg backwards until it is in slight hyperextension. Hold briefly and control it back to the starting position. Alternate legs after each set.

Variation: Execute with hands on hips for balance.

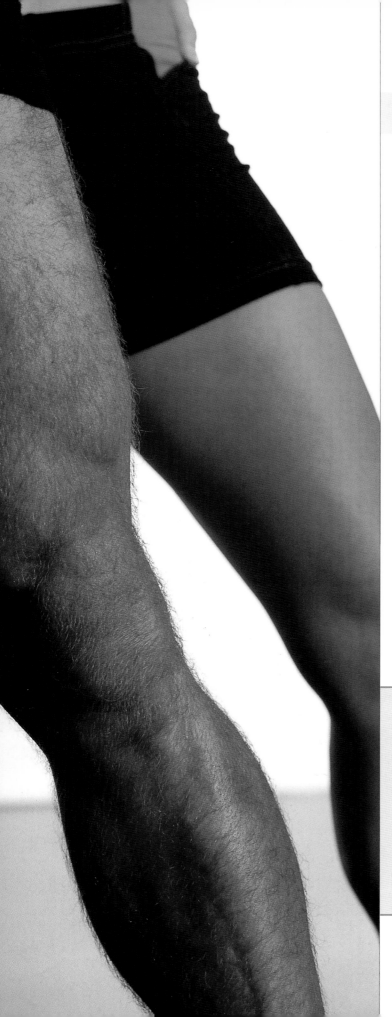

Thighs

▼ Incline leg press

Classification: Core. **Primary muscles:** Quadriceps, gluteus maximus.

Starting position: Lie back on the seat with your lower back firmly against the backrest. Place your feet shoulder width apart on the foot platform, with your feet slightly turned out. Grasp the handles of the incline leg press, release the stoppers and take the load on your legs.

Execution: Bend your legs and control the weight with your knees moving towards your chest. Allow your knees to flex a little more than 90°, until your thighs and the foot platform are almost parallel. Slowly extend your legs and push the platform back to its starting position. Keep your knees slightly bent throughout.

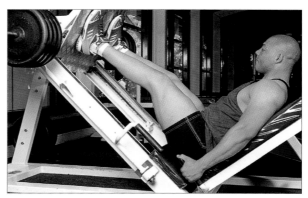

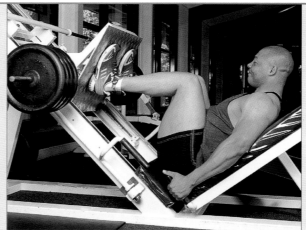

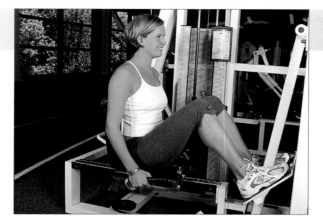
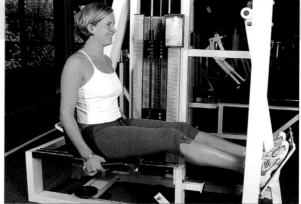

▲ Seated leg press

Classification: Core. **Primary muscles:** Quadriceps, gluteus maximus.

Starting position: Sit with your lower back firmly against the backrest of the leg press. Place your feet on the foot-plates with your toes slightly turned out. Make sure your knee angle is a little less than 90°.

Execution: Grasp the handles and extend your legs. Do not lock them. Bend your legs and control the weight downwards with your knees moving towards your chest. Lower the weight stack until it nearly touches the remaining weights and push your legs back to the extended position.

! ▼ Forward lunge

Classification: Auxiliary. **Primary muscles:** Quadriceps, gluteus maximus, hamstrings.

Starting position: Stand with the barbell supported on your shoulders and your hands grasping it with an overhand grip, shoulder width apart. Keep the feet at the same distance.

Execution: Keeping your back straight and your torso upright, lunge forward with the right leg. Bend this leg until about 90°, with the left leg 5–10cm (2–4in) above the ground. Push back with the right leg and return in one movement to the starting position. Alternate legs.

Variations: Execute with dumbbells; side lunge.

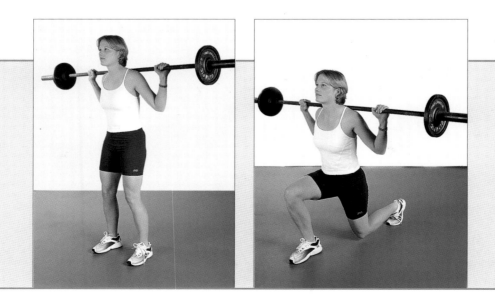

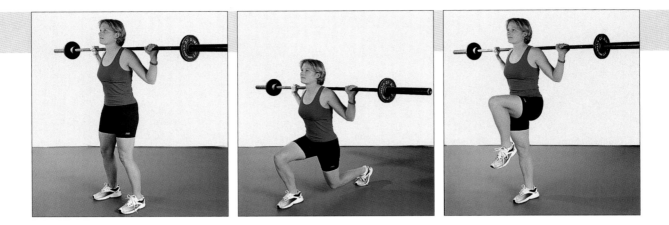

! ▲ Crane lunge

Classification: Auxiliary. **Primary muscles:** Quadriceps, gluteus maximus, hamstrings.

Starting position: Stand with the barbell supported on your shoulders, grasping the bar with an overhand grip, hands shoulder width apart. Keep the feet at the same distance.

Execution: Keeping the back straight and torso upright, lunge forward with your right leg. Bend this leg until about 90°, with your left leg 5–10cm (2–4in) above the ground. Push up and forward with your right leg and follow through with your left leg, until the right leg is extended and the left knee is lifted in the crane position. Lower the left leg to the trailing position and return to the starting position. Alternate legs.

Variation: Execute with dumbbells.

▼ Step-up

Classification: Auxiliary. **Primary muscles:** Quadriceps, gluteus maximus, hamstrings.

Starting position: Stand facing the bench with the barbell supported on your shoulders, grasping the bar with an overhand grip, hands shoulder width apart. Keep the feet at the same distance.

Execution: Keeping the back straight and torso upright, step onto the bench with your right leg. Push and extend the right leg and lift the body and left leg onto the bench. Step down with the right leg and then down with the left leg to the starting position. Alternate leading legs.

Variations: Step-up in a crane position (*see crane lunge*); execute with dumbbells.

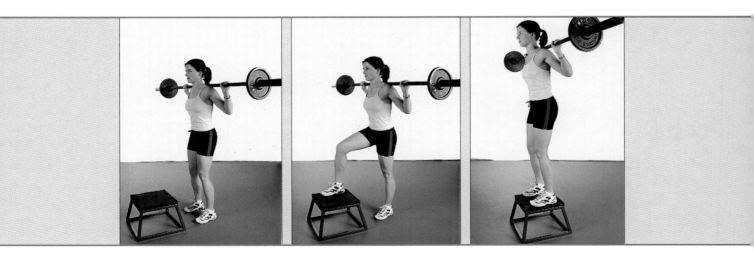

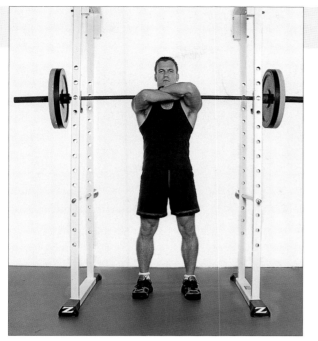

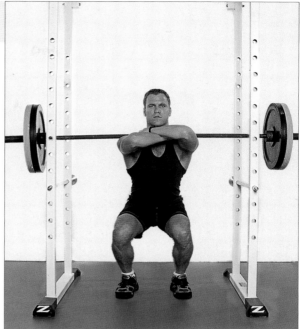

! ▲ Front squat

Classification: Structural. **Primary muscles:** Quadriceps, hamstrings, gluteus maximus.

Starting position: Stand with the barbell supported across your collarbones and anterior shoulders. Flex your arms and cross them over the bar. Hold it steady with an open grip and elbows high (1). Keep your feet about shoulder width apart and slightly turned out. Keep the lower back slightly arched and your torso leaning forward.

Execution: Keeping your head up and your torso stationary throughout, flex first in the knees and then in the hips and lower the body until the thighs are parallel to the floor. Side view (2) shows depth of squat. Push and extend the knees and hips upwards, without losing posture, back to the starting position. Always allow the knees to travel aligned over the feet.

Variation: Execute with closed overhand grip, hands shoulder width apart.

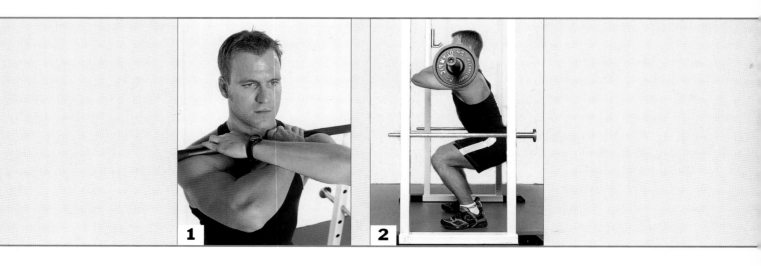

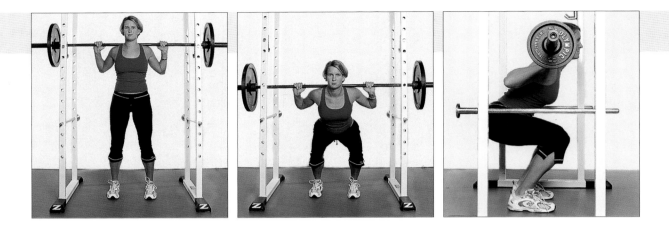

! ▲ Back squat

Classification: Structural. **Primary muscles:** Quadriceps, hamstrings, gluteus maximus.

Starting position: Stand with the barbell supported behind your head at the base of your neck, grasping the bar with an overhand grip, hands shoulder width apart. Keep your feet at the same distance and slightly turned out. Keep your lower back arched and keep your torso leaning forwards.

Execution: Keeping your head up and your torso sta-tionary throughout, flex first in the knees and then in the hips, and lower your body until your thighs are parallel to the floor (side view shows depth of squat). Push and extend your knees and hips upwards, without losing your posture, back to the starting position. Always allow the knees to travel aligned over the feet.

Variations: Low-bar position; Smith Machine squat.

▼ Prone leg curl

Classification: Auxiliary. **Primary muscles:** Hamstrings.

Starting position: Lie prone on the curl machine with your ankles under the footpads. Grasp the handles provided for support. Keep your head and upper body down against the curl bench throughout.

Execution: Curl the legs in as far towards the buttocks as possible. Hold briefly and return to the starting position.

Variations: Single leg; standing leg curl.

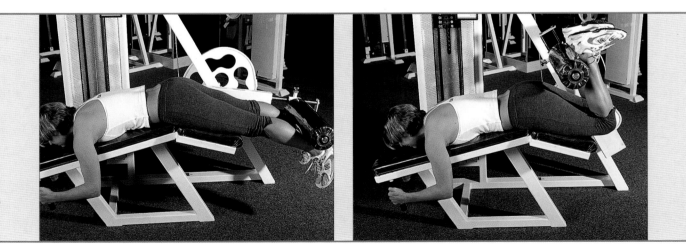

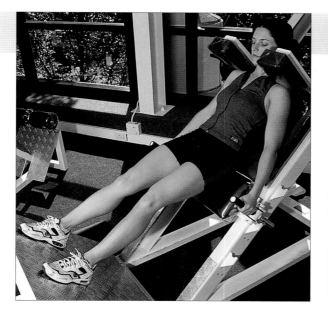

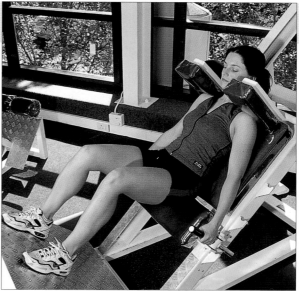

▲ Hack squat

Classification: Core. **Primary muscles:** Quadriceps, hamstrings, gluteus maximus.

Starting position: Stand with the hack-squat machine's shoulder pads on your shoulders and back pressed firmly against the backrest. Keep your feet shoulder width apart against the angled platform and slightly turned out.

Execution: Flex in the knees and hips, and lower your body until your hip and knee angles are at approximately 90°. Push and extend the knees and hips upwards. Always allow the knees to travel aligned over the feet.

▼ Machine leg extension

Classification: Auxiliary. **Primary muscles:** Quadriceps.

Starting position: Sit with your back pressed firmly against the backrest, the shin pad against the front of your ankles and the back of your knees against the seat's edge. Grasp the handles at the sides of the seat.

Execution: Without using the hips to assist you, extend your legs by lifting the lever arm upwards until your legs are straight. Hold briefly and control back to the starting position.

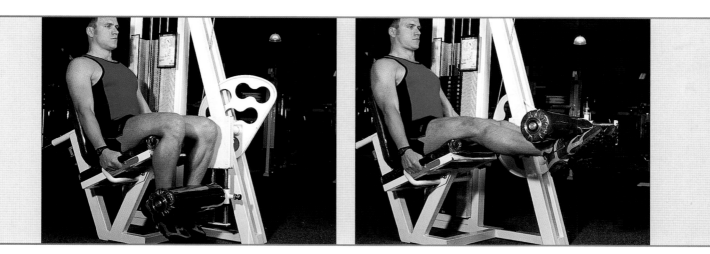

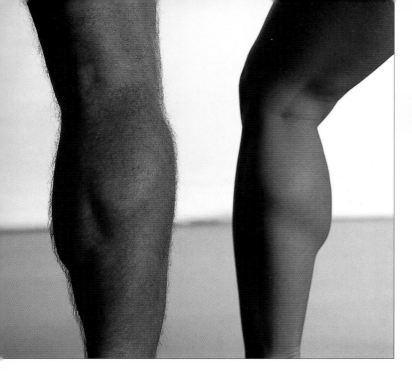

Lower legs and feet

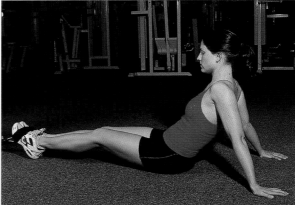

▼ Standing calf raise

Classification: Auxiliary. **Primary muscles:** Soleus, gastrocnemius.

Starting position: Stand under the shoulder pads with only the balls of your feet on the elevated foot platform. Grab the handles provided for stability. Keep the knees slightly bent throughout and your toes pointing straight ahead.

Execution: Slowly lower your heels as far as you can go. Push upwards and lift the heels as high as possible.

Variations: Execute with toes pointing in or out; single-leg calf raise.

◆ Seated cable pull

Classification: Auxiliary. **Primary muscles:** Tibialis anterior.

Starting position: Sit on the floor facing the low pulley with your legs extended in front of you, knees slightly bent. Place the ankle strap over the bridges of your feet and tighten its grip. Sit away from the pulley to tension the cable, knees still bent.

Execution: Using your feet, pull the cable as far in towards your shins as possible. Hold briefly and control back to the starting position.

Variations: Single leg; eversion (external rotation); inversion (internal rotation).

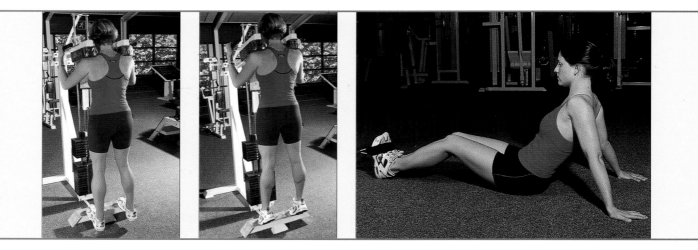

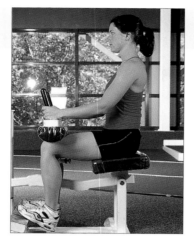 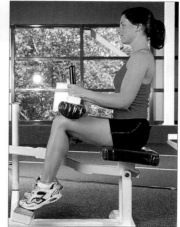

▲ Seated machine calf raise

Classification: Auxiliary. **Primary muscles:** Soleus.

Starting position: Sit on the machine with only the balls of your feet on the elevated foot platform and the knee pads resting on your knees. Grab the handles provided for stability. Keep your toes pointing straight ahead. Unhook the safety stop.

Execution: Slowly lower your heels as far as they can go. Push upwards and lift the heels as high as possible.

Variations: Execute with toes pointing in or out; single-leg calf raise.

! ▼ Donkey calf raise

Classification: Auxiliary. **Primary muscles:** Soleus, gastrocnemius.

Starting position: Stand on a step with only the balls of the feet on the edge of it. Bend forward in the hips until your torso is parallel to the floor. Stabilize your body against the flat bench in front of you. Keep your toes pointing straight ahead. Allow a training partner to straddle over your back and hips. Keep your knees slightly bent throughout.

Execution: Slowly lower the heels as far as they can go. Push upwards and lift the heels as high as possible.

Variation: Execute with toes pointing in or out.

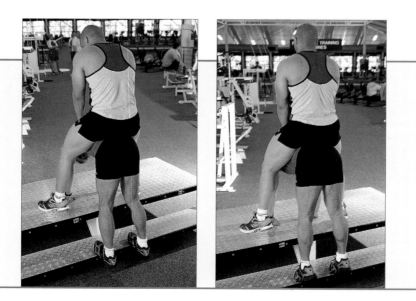

Total body and power

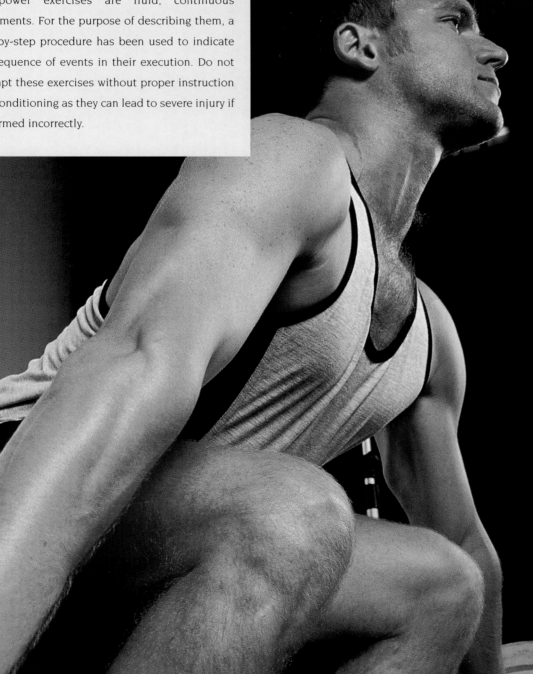

All power exercises are fluid, continuous movements. For the purpose of describing them, a step-by-step procedure has been used to indicate the sequence of events in their execution. Do not attempt these exercises without proper instruction and conditioning as they can lead to severe injury if performed incorrectly.

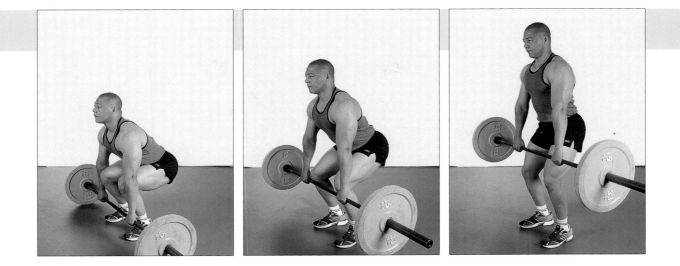

! High pull

Classification: Power (caution – perform under supervision until proficient). **Primary muscles:** Total body.

Starting position: Stand with your feet more or less shoulder width apart, feet under the bar. Grasp the bar using a hooked, overhand grip with your hands also approximately shoulder width apart. Slightly arch the lower back, push the buttocks out, the shoulders back, and lift the head.

Execution: Keep the bar close to the body at all times.

Explosively thrust it upwards using the legs and lower back. Once it reaches mid-thigh level, thrust the hips forwards and accelerate it upwards. Additionally, use the shoulders and upper back to assist, bend the elbows and pull with the arms to further accelerate the bar, until it reaches shoulder height. Control the bar back down to the thighs and then lower it to the ground.

Variations: High pull with a snatch-grip; hang pull (*see hang clean p99*).

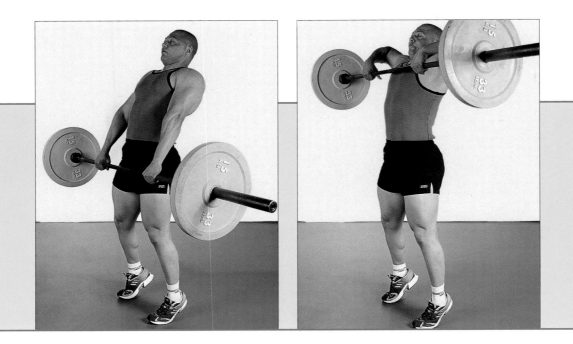

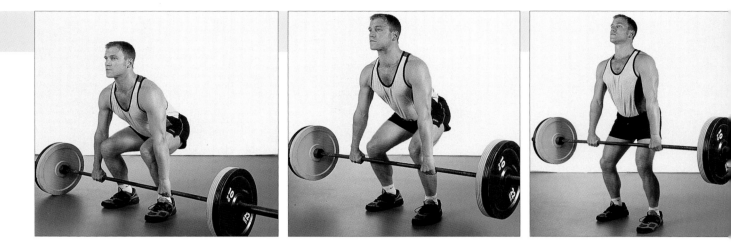

! Power clean

Classification: Power (caution – perform under super-vision until proficient). **Primary muscles:** Total body.

Starting position: Stand with your feet more or less shoulder width apart and under the bar, shins touching. Grasp the bar using a hooked, overhand grip with your hands slightly wider than shoulder width apart. Arch the lower back a little, push the buttocks out, pull the shoulders back, and lift the head.

Execution: Keep the bar close to the body at all times. Explosively thrust it upwards using your legs and lower back. Once the bar reaches mid-thigh level, thrust the hips forwards and accelerate the bar. Additionally, use the shoulders, upper back and arm muscles to assist. Bend the elbows and, as the bar moves past navel height, pull the body underneath the accelerating bar and rotate the arms under it, drop into a quarter-squat position and catch it on the upper chest and shoulders with your elbows high. Stand up and stabilize. Control the bar back down to the thighs and then lower it back to the ground.

Variations: Hang clean; clean-and-jerk (combination of the power clean and the push jerk).

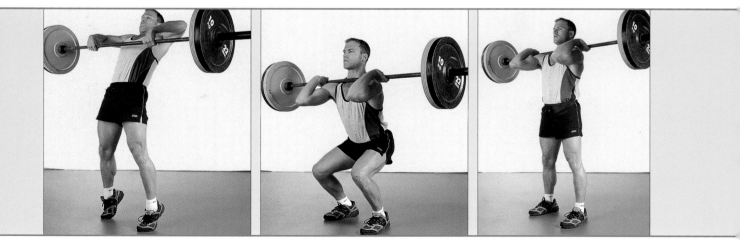

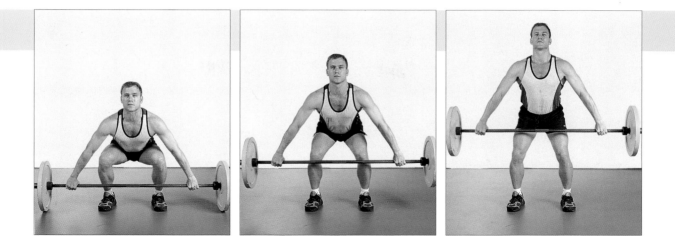

! Power snatch

Classification: Power (caution – perform under supervision until proficient). **Primary muscles:** Total body.

Starting position: Stand with your feet more or less shoulder width apart and under the bar, shins touching. Grasp the bar using a hooked, overhand grip and keep your hands wide apart (insert shows measurement of exact distance). Slightly arch your lower back, push the buttocks out, pull the shoulders back and lift the head.

Execution: Keep the bar close to the body at all times. Explosively thrust it upwards using the muscles of the legs and lower back. Once the bar reaches mid-thigh level, thrust the hips forwards and accelerate it up. During this movement, assist the bar upwards using the

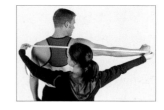

shoulder and upper back muscles, bend the elbows and continue to pull it upwards until it reaches approximately shoulder height. As the bar continues moving upwards, pull the body underneath the bar and rotate the arms under it, drop into a quarter-squat position, extend the arms and catch the bar overhead with fully outstretched arms and the bar slightly behind the head. Stand up and stabilize. Control the bar back down to the thighs and then lower it to the ground.

Variation: Hang snatch.

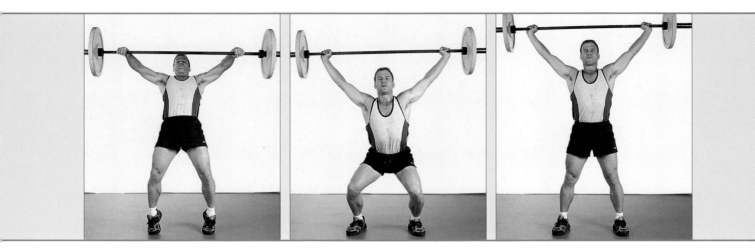

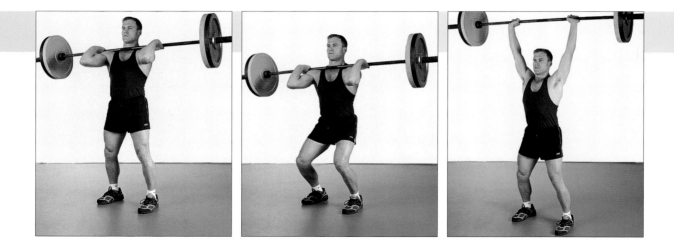

! ▲ Push jerk

Classification: Power (caution – perform under supervision until proficient). **Primary muscles:** Total body.

Starting position: Stand erect with feet shoulder width apart, feet slightly turned out and the barbell resting on the front of your shoulders. Hold the bar with a closed overhand grip, your hands also shoulder width apart.

Execution: Using a small movement, rapidly dip downwards in the knees and hips, reverse direction and push the barbell to an extended position overhead, using a forceful extension of your hips, knees and ankles to assist you.

Variations: Push press (which uses less assistance from the hips and knees); split jerk; plyometric push jerk.

! ▼ Jump squat

Classification: Power (caution – perform under supervision until proficient). **Primary muscles:** Quadriceps, hamstrings, gluteus maximus.

Starting position: Start in an upright position in a Smith Machine holding the bar tightly against the base of your neck with a narrow grip. In this way the bar is supported against the trapezius muscles and will not separate from the body during jumping. Alternatively, use a harness.

Execution: Maintaining the same criteria as for back squats, dip rapidly into a half-squat position and explosively jump upwards as high as you can. This can either be done as single repetitions or you can land and take off again in one continuous movement.

Variation: Plyometric split squat.

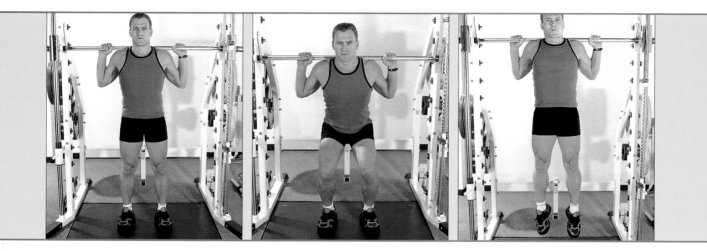

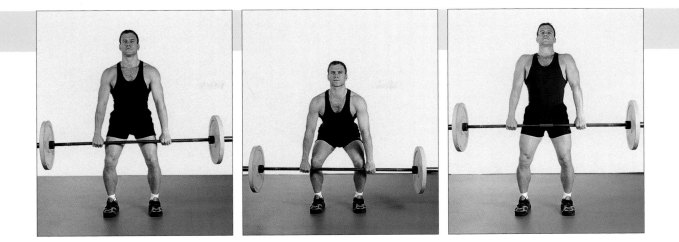

! Hang clean

Classification: Power (caution – perform under super-vision until proficient). **Primary muscles:** Total upper body.

Starting position: Stand with your feet more or less shoulder width apart and under the bar, shins touching. Grasp the bar using a hooked, overhand grip with your hands slightly wider than shoulder width apart. Slightly arch the lower back, push the buttocks out, pull the shoulders back, and lift the head. Lift the bar until it hangs stationary in front of the thighs, just above the knees.

Execution: Keep the bar close to the body at all times. Dip slightly and explosively thrust it upwards. Once the bar reaches mid-thigh level, thrust the hips forwards and accelerate the bar upwards. Additionally, use the shoulders, upper back and arm muscles to assist. As the bar moves past navel height, bend the elbows and pull the body underneath the accelerating bar and rotate the arms under it, drop into a quarter-squat position and catch it on the upper chest and shoulders with your elbows high. Stand up and stabilize. Control the bar back down to the thighs and starting position.

Variations: Hang snatch; hang pull; from block support.

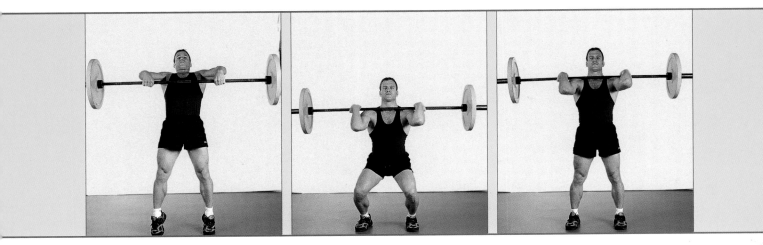

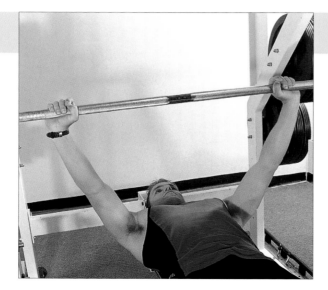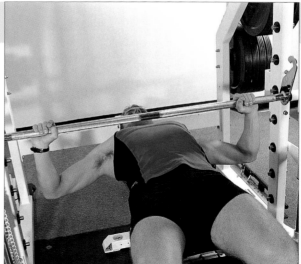

! **Rebound bench throw**

Classification: Power (caution – perform under supervision until proficient). **Primary muscles:** Pectoralis major (middle), anterior deltoid, triceps.

Starting position: Adjust the safety stoppers on the Smith Machine so that the bar will not land on your chest if it is missed. Use an overhand closed grip with your hands 7–10cm (3–4in) wider than shoulder width apart. Your feet should either be placed on the floor, shoulder width apart, on the bench or lifted in the air. Lift the bar off its supports and extend the arms upwards.

Execution: Rapidly lower the bar towards the nipple line. Quickly reverse direction and explosively push the bar upwards and release it. This exercise can either be done as individual repetitions, or subsequently catch it and rapidly throw it again in one movement.

Variation: Rebound incline bench throw.

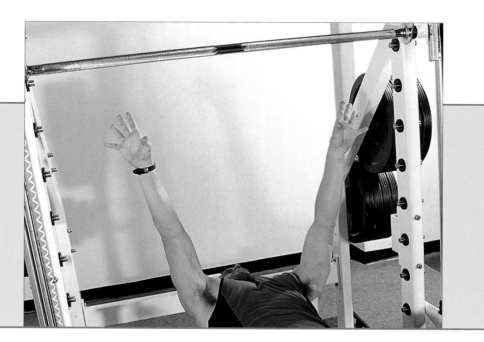

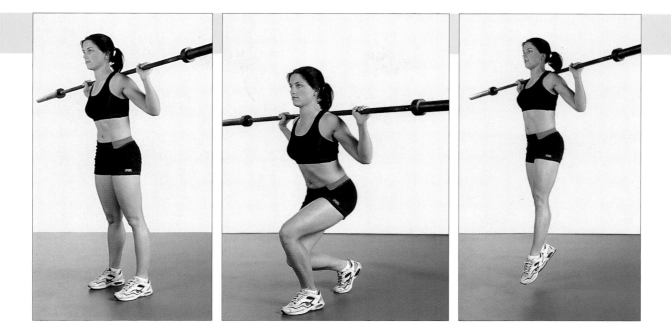

! ▲ Reverse lunge

Classification: Power (caution – perform under supervision until proficient). **Primary muscles:** Quadriceps, gluteus maximus, hamstrings.

Starting position: Stand with the barbell supported on your shoulders, and your hands grasping the bar shoulder width apart in an overhand grip. Also keep the feet shoulder width apart.

Execution: Keeping your back straight and your torso upright, take a small stride backwards with your right leg. Rapidly bend the left leg until it is about 90°, with your right knee 5–10cm (2–4in) above the ground. Push with both legs and explosively jump upwards, landing on both feet in the starting position. Alternate legs.

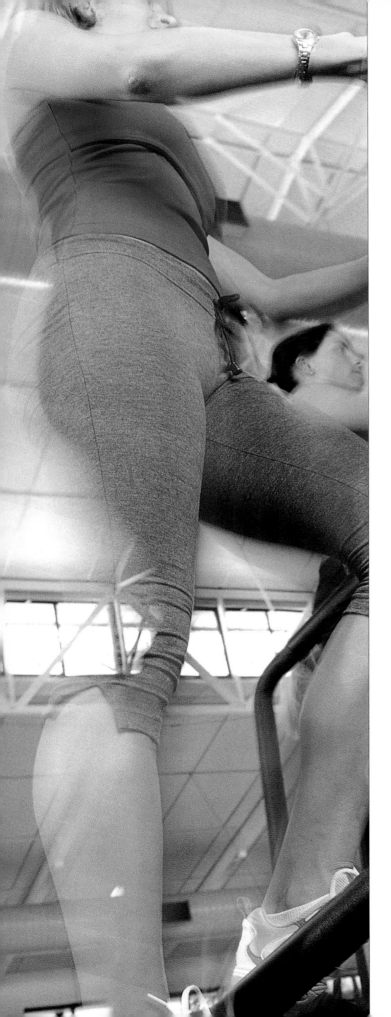

Methods of weight training

When resistance-training programmes

are prescribed, certain basic variables

are adapted to the needs, goals and

body type of the individual. The main

variables are: load/resistance, repetitions,

rest periods and sets.

This chapter, together with sample

programmes, will indicate ways in which

these variables can be manipulated to

achieve the following goals: weight loss,

cardiovascular endurance,

muscle endurance, muscle tone,

hypertrophy, strength, and power.

Load/resistance

The load with which to train depends on your goal and your present level of conditioning. The basic guidelines are that light loads are for endurance training and heavy loads for strength training. When selecting a load, and for purposes of monitoring your improvement, you need to test for a reference marker. This is usually the maximum load that you can lift correctly only once through a complete range of motion in a specific exercise. This is known as your maximal strength or 1RM (one-repetition maximum). Measuring directly for 1RM is not always practical, due to factors such as your training background, the nature of the muscles being tested (smaller muscle groups are put at greater risk of injury), your susceptibility to fatigue, and your risk of injury due to other factors. For these reasons it may be necessary to predict 1RM by, for example, first determining your 10RM (maximum weight that can be lifted 10 times with good form), and

TRAINING GOAL VERSUS LOAD	
Training goal	**Range of loads using %1RM**
Weight loss	40–60%1RM
Cardiovascular endurance	50–70%1RM
Muscle endurance	30–80%1RM
Muscle tone	60–75%1RM
Hypertrophy	70–85%1RM
Strength	80–100%1RM
Power	30–90%1RM

then calculating your 1RM with the aid of various conversion tables and formulae (not provided in this book).

You will usually train at a percentage of 1RM. In the case of 75%1RM, for instance, if your 1RM were 100kg (or, for purposes of easy calculation, assume a 1RM of 100 lb),

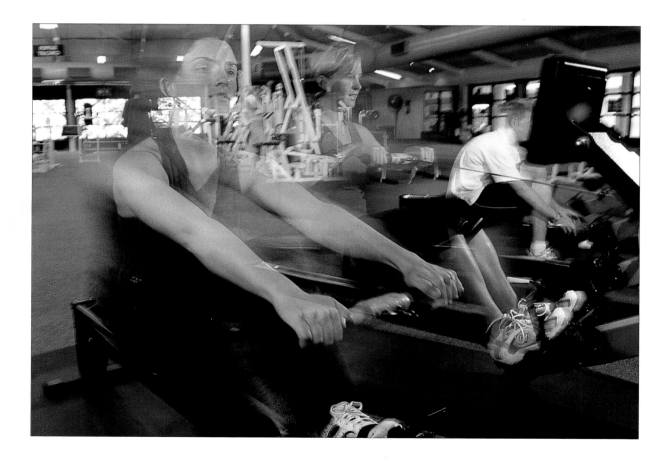

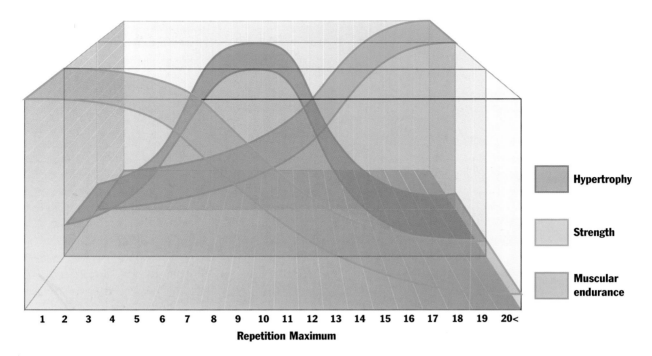

1 2 3 4 5 6 7 8 9 10 11 12 13 14 15 16 17 18 19 20<

Repetition Maximum

The ranges of loads, which are optimal for the training goals of strength, hypertrophy and muscle endurance.

you would be training with a 75kg (or 75 lb) load. Predicted 1RM is slightly less accurate than the direct method of establishing 1RM, but is good enough to monitor performance and act as a reference marker. For large muscle groups or core exercises, such as the incline leg press and bench press, you can test directly for 1RM. However, when selecting loads for smaller muscle groups or assistance exercises such as bicep curls and lateral raises, the risk of injury makes the indirect method preferable.

Whatever method is used to determine 1RM, you choose your training load according to your training goal.

Repetitions

Repetitions and load have an inverse relationship. The heavier the weight, the fewer repetitions can be performed. The inappropriate number of repetitions will reduce your chances of reaching your goal. For example, if you are power training and do too many repetitions in a set, you risk losing form and explosiveness due to fatigue. You will miss the purpose of the exercise, which is developing power – not muscle endurance.

TRAINING GOAL VERSUS REPETITIONS

Training goal	Repetitions
Weight loss	15–30 reps
Cardiovascular endurance	12–25 reps
Muscle endurance	12–30 reps
Muscle toning	12–15 reps
Hypertrophy	6–12 reps
Strength	1–8 reps
Power	1–6 reps

Rest periods

The rest periods between sets and exercises are determined by the loads, repetitions and the training goals of each programme. Generally, the heavier the load, the longer the rest period between sets, and the lighter the load, the shorter the rest period. The rules of rest-period manipulation depend on the muscle groups involved and the weight used, which does not have to be uniform for all muscle groups in a training session. The range of rest periods should only be used as a guideline.

TRAINING GOAL VERSUS REST PERIODS	
Training goal	Rest periods between sets
Weight loss	15–30sec
Cardiovascular endurance	15–60sec
Muscle endurance	30sec–2min
Muscle toning	30sec–2min
Hypertrophy	30–90sec
Strength	2–8min
Power	2–8min

TRAINING GOAL VERSUS NUMBER OF SETS	
Training goal	Sets
Weight loss	1–2 sets
Cardiovascular endurance	1–3 sets
Muscle endurance	2–3 sets
Muscle toning	2–3 sets
Hypertrophy	4–6 sets
Strength	4–5 sets
Power	4–5 sets

Sets

Sets are selected according to the load, training goal and number of repetitions. As a rule of thumb, if you do fewer repetitions you can do more sets. However, the time you have available for training is also an important factor to consider. If you are, for example, doing 30 repetitions of an exercise, it can take a long time to perform four to five sets and it can induce fatigue. It will also limit your time available for other exercises, and thus deter you from training effectively.

It is best not to stay with one routine for long. Consult a professional on how to vary your training. You need a specific, structured and periodized training plan, which breaks down your ultimate training goal into smaller, more reachable interim goals. This will help you focus on short-term results while working towards a long-term goal. Vary training in a progressive manner to prevent overtraining or stagnation.

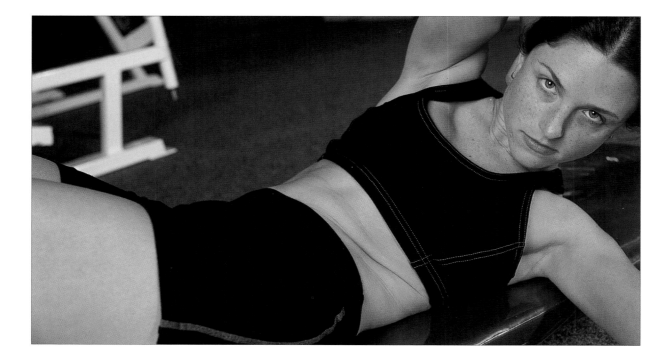

Exercise programmes

Weight loss

A weight-loss programme should focus on losing body fat rather than body mass. Body mass may even increase slightly at first due to increased muscle mass, which is more dense (weighs more) than fat. People who go on a weight-loss programme have usually been inactive for some time, so their muscles respond quickly. Once their bodies adapt to the stresses put on them, this initial increase in body mass plateaus and, if they continue with the programme, body-mass decreases over time.

Many weight-loss programmes focus on **low-intensity endurance activities.** This is partly because most people on weight-loss programmes cannot maintain higher intensities. However, the main reason is that during low-intensity endurance exercise body fat is the main source of energy. However, **interval training** (work intervals separated by rest intervals) develops your recovery fitness and allows for a greater work rate during a session than would be possible if the same exercise were performed continuously. It may also result in expending more 'fat calories' than continuous low-intensity exercise.

If, for argument's sake, 80% of calories expended during a low-intensity endurance workout are from fat sources and you burn 200 calories in a session, you would have burnt 160 'fat calories' during that time.

Let's say you undertake a session of interval training at a higher intensity, and you burn a total of 300 calories, of which 65% are derived from fat sources. You will burn more 'fat calories' (195) than in the low-intensity endurance exercise example, even though the percentage contribution from fat sources is less.

INCREASE RESTING METABOLISM

For weight loss, there are also advantages to stimulating and developing your muscles through resistance training.

By activating them on a regular basis and increasing your muscle mass, you can increase your resting metabolism, thereby burning more energy during rest, albeit not to a major extent.

A big problem with weight-loss programmes is boredom and a resulting loss of interest. The antidote is to vary your training. Circuit training is an excellent form of interval training and is a great way to stimulate weight loss. Circuit training alternates upper-body and lower-body exercises that progress from large to small muscle groups for optimal training. The loads are usually between 40 and 60%1RM. Most gyms use a 45-second work interval separated by a 15-second recovery interval. Others have a 30-second work interval and a 30-second recovery interval.

You can start with a circuit routine that lasts about 20 minutes (warm-up excluded). As you become fitter, you can increase your number of circuits and the duration of exercise. A more advanced form of circuit training is the super-circuit. This alternates resistance exercises with other forms of exercise. For the purposes of weight loss an aerobic exercise should be added between each weight-training exercise. For example, a rowing exercise can be inserted between the machine bench press and leg press, or cycling between the leg press and seated vertical row.

BEGINNER'S WEIGHT-LOSS PROGRAMME

The key objective of this programme is to initiate a lifestyle change. The focus is less on the volume of training and more on participation and variation of regimens, using major muscle groups in a circuit fashion. Beat boredom by varying your exercises and varying the order of the exercises regularly.

INTERMEDIATE PROGRAMME

For this programme, the focus moves to combining aerobic activities with resistance-training in a super-circuit fashion. After this, you can advance to the cardiovascular programme.

AN EXAMPLE OF A BEGINNER'S WEIGHT-LOSS PROGRAMME

No.	Exercise	Load (%1RM)	Sets	Reps	Rest
1	Warm-up on stationary bicycle or treadmill, and stretch (±12–15min)	N/A	N/A	N/A	1–2min
2	Bench press machine	40–50%	1–2	15–20	15–30sec
3	Abdominal crunch	N/A	1–2	10–15	15–30sec
4	Lat pulldown	40–50%	1–2	15–20	15–30sec
5	Seated leg press	40–50%	1–2	15–20	15–30sec
6	Machine flye	40–50%	1–2	15–20	15–30sec
7	Hanging leg raise (bent knee)	N/A	1–2	10–15	15–30sec
8	Seated cable row	40–50%	1–2	15–20	15–30sec
9	Leg extension	40–50%	1–2	15–20	15–30sec
10	Machine shoulder press	40–50%	1–2	15–20	15–30sec
11	Prone leg curl	40–50%	1–2	15–20	15–30sec
12	Machine bicep curl	40–50%	1–2	15–20	15–30sec
13	Abdominal crunch	N/A	1–2	10–15	15–30sec
14	Tricep pressdown	40–50%	1–2	15–20	15–30sec
15	Cool-down on stationary bicycle or treadmill (±5–10min)	N/A	N/A	N/A	N/A

Comments: After the warm-up, perform exercises 2 to 14 continuously in a circuit format. Only complete one circuit. Perform this workout twice a week. During the remainder of the week include additional cardiovascular activities such as walking, cycling or swimming, for optimal results. Progress gradually to two circuits.

AN EXAMPLE OF AN INTERMEDIATE WEIGHT-LOSS PROGRAMME

No.	Exercise	Load (%1RM)	Sets	Reps	Rest
1	Warm-up on stationary bicycle or treadmill, and stretch (±12–15min)	N/A	N/A	N/A	1–2min
2	Machine chest press	50–60%	2	20–30	15–30sec
3	Seated leg press	50–60%	2	20–30	15–30sec
4	Cycling*	N/A	1	N/A	15–30sec
5	Rowing torso machine	50–60%	2	20–30	15–30sec
6	Machine crunch	50–60%	2	20–30	15–30sec
7	Rowing ergometer *	N/A	1	N/A	15–30sec
8	Machine leg extension	50–60%	2	20–30	15–30sec
9	Machine flye	50–60%	2	20–30	15–30sec
10	Stair-climber *	N/A	1	N/A	15–30sec
11	Twist-crunch	50–60%	2	8–10 per side	15–30sec
12	Prone leg curl	50–60%	2	20–30	15–30sec
13	Treadmill *	N/A	1	N/A	15–30sec
14	Standing cable bicep curl	50–60%	2	20–30	15–30sec
15	Seated calf raise	50–60%	2	20–30	15–30sec
16	Cool-down on stationary bicycle or treadmill (±5–10min)	N/A	N/A	N/A	N/A

Comments: * Indicates two intervals, usually to a total of about 2 minutes.
After the warm-up, do exercises 2 to 15 continuously in a circuit format. Do one set of each until all the exercises have been done. Complete the second circuit as indicated. Do this workout two to three times a week. During the remainder of the week include cardiovascular activities such as walking, cycling or swimming.

Cardiovascular endurance

Cardiovascular endurance is increased by overloading the heart-and-lung system sufficiently to increase your heart and breathing rates during exercise. Your heart rate will increase according to the intensity of the exercise, as will your breathing rate – to vent the build-up of carbon dioxide in the blood. Your heart rate can be used to gauge the intensity of a cardiovascular-endurance exercise. Your maximal heart rate (MHR) can be predicted using the equation: MHR = 220 minus your age. The formula has an error of about 10%. For a more accurate gauge of your maximum heart rate, consult a fitness or medical professional.

For cardiovascular endurance you want to train at 70–90% of your maximum heart rate to tax your heart-lung system sufficiently. To ensure that you are training in your zone, you need to measure your heart rate during exercise. You could either take your pulse (counting the number of heart beats in 15 seconds and multiplying by four) or, preferably, use a heart-rate monitor.

The cardiovascular-endurance programme is similar to the weight-loss programme, except that you would start with a higher load and exercise intensity, and your training sessions would be longer. For optimal cardiovascular improvement you should, however, undertake regular aerobic training such as distance running or cycling.

Regular aerobic training is generally better than circuit training for development of cardiovascular endurance, although the latter provides overall body and muscle development. Circuit and super-circuit training should be used as a form of cross training for cardiovascular endurance and not as a main form of training for this goal.

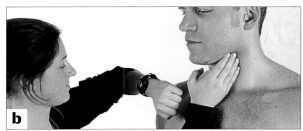

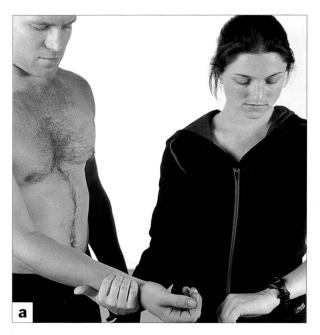

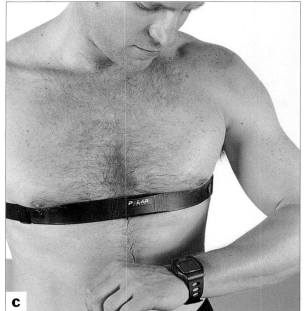

(a) Heart rate can be measured at the radial pulse (on the thumb side of the inner wrist).

(b) The carotid pulse is next to the air passage.

In both cases it is necessary to stand still and take the pulse immediately because movement and delay can influence the accuracy of the measurement.

(c) A heart-rate monitor is the most accurate.

AN EXAMPLE OF AN INTERMEDIATE CARDIOVASCULAR PROGRAMME

No.	Exercise	Load (%1RM)	Sets	Reps	Rest
1	Warm-up on stationary bicycle or tread-mill, and stretch (±12–15min)	N/A	N/A	N/A	1–2min
2	Machine bench press	60–70%	2	12–15	15–30sec
3*	Cycling	N/A	2	N/A	15–30sec
4	Seated vertical row	60–70%	2	12–15	15–30sec
5*	Treadmill	N/A	2	N/A	15–30sec
6	Seated leg press	60–70%	2	15–20	15–30sec
7*	Rowing ergometer	N/A	2	N/A	15–30sec
8	Hanging leg-raise	N/A	2	15-20	15–30sec
9*	Stair-climber	N/A	2	N/A	15–30sec
10	Machine shoulder press	60–70%	2	12–15	15–30sec
11*	Elliptic cycle	N/A	2	N/A	15–30sec
12	Lat pulldown	60–70%	2	12–15	15–30sec
13*	Rope-skipping	N/A	2	N/A	15–30sec
14	Standing tricep pressdown	60–70%	2	12–15	15–30sec
15*	Bench step-up	N/A	2	N/A	15–30sec
16	Machine bicep curl	60–70%	2	12–15	15–30sec
17	Cool-down on stationary bicycle or treadmill (±5–10min)	N/A	N/A	N/A	N/A

Comments: *Sufficient intensity to raise heart rate to target values.
After the warm-up, perform exercises 2 to16 continuously in a circuit format. Maintain a heart rate of between 70 and 85% of MHR throughout. Perform this workout two to three times a week. During the remainder of the week include additional cardiovascular activities for optimal results.

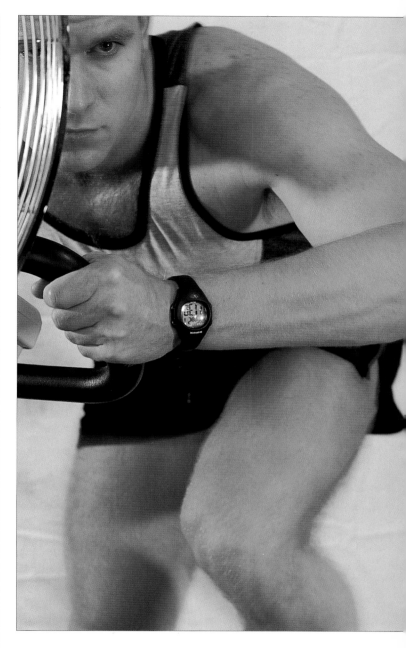

The **Karvonen equation** is another method of gauging exercise intensity during cardiovascular exercise. This equation takes a further variable into account, namely heart rate reserve (HRR). This is the difference between your resting and maximum heart rates. It uses a percentage of heart rate reserve (HRR) added to your resting heart rate (RHR) to determine target heart rate (THR).

THR = RHR + % of (MHR - RHR)

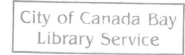

AN EXAMPLE OF AN ADVANCED CARDIOVASCULAR PROGRAMME

No.	Exercise	Load (%1RM)	Sets	Reps	Rest	No.	Exercise	Load (%1RM)	Sets	Reps	Rest
1	Warm-up on stationary bicycle or treadmill, and stretch (±12–15min)	N/A	N/A	N/A	1–2min	12	Rowing ergometer	N/A	2	N/A	15–30sec
						13	Bench step-up	N/A	1	45sec	15–30sec
2	Machine chest press	70%	2	12–15	15–30sec	14	Military press	70%	2	12–15	15–30sec
						15	Treadmill	N/A	2	N/A	15–30sec
3	Treadmill	N/A	2	N/A	15–30sec	16	Cycling	N/A	1	N/A	15–30sec
4	Rowing ergometer	N/A	1	N/A	15–30sec	17	Chin-up	N/A	2	Max	15–30sec
5	Standing tricep pressdown	70%	2	12–15	15–30sec	18	Stair-climber	N/A	2	N/A	15–30sec
6	Cycling	N/A	2	N/A	15–30sec	19	Elliptic cycle	N/A	1	N/A	15–30sec
7	Stair-climber	N/A	1	N/A	15–30sec	20	Preacher curl	70%	2	12–15	15–30sec
8	Seated leg press	70%	2	12–15	15–30sec	21	Hanging leg-raise	N/A	2	20–25	15–30sec
9	Bench step-up	N/A	2	45sec	15–30sec	22	Cool-down on stationary bicycle or treadmill (±5-10min)	N/A	N/A	N/A	N/A
10	Elliptic cycle	N/A	1	N/A	15–30sec						
11	Machine leg extension	70%	2	12–15	15–30sec						

Comments: After the warm-up, perform exercises 2 to 21 continuously in a circuit format. Maintain a heart rate of between 80 and 90% of MHR throughout. Perform this workout 2–3 times a week. During the remainder of the week include additional cardiovascular activities such as jogging, cycling or swimming for optimal results.

For development of cardiovascular endurance you need to focus on large muscle groups, a relatively low load and short rest periods. It takes about 12 to 15 minutes for the cardiovascular system to get up and running properly, so you need to train for at least 45 minutes, which includes your warm-up and cool-down session.

An aerobic super-circuit, where your resistance is between 50 and 70%1RM and your heart rate between 70 and 90% of MHR throughout, should yield optimal results from a resistance-training perspective. By combining aerobic activities with resistance training, as in the aerobic super-circuit, you will increase the cardiovascular benefits.

INTERMEDIATE PROGRAMME

(Beginners can start with an intermediate weight-loss programme.) The aim of this programme is to elevate your heart rate to between 70 and 85% of MHR with the focus on higher intensity and shorter rest periods.

ADVANCED PROGRAMME

The key is elevating the heart rate to between 80 and 90% of MHR. Therefore, the focus is on increasing training intensity and incorporating increased aerobic intervals. Different aerobic activities, as with the previous programmes, indicate options for the aerobic intervals.

Muscle endurance

Muscle endurance can mean two things: either sustaining a contraction for as long as possible, namely holding a weight until failure, or performing as many repetitions as possible with a specific weight.

The average person can develop muscle endurance from general strength training. Work capacity also improves with strength. This can be illustrated by asking two people to perform as many push-ups as possible. The stronger of the two will do the most push-ups. The reason for this is that for the stronger person, the effort of pushing up body mass is less.

For more specific muscle endurance you can train between 50 and 70%1RM, performing 12 to 20 repetitions and resting 30 to 60 seconds between sets and exercises. This format is considered the most effective in developing overall muscle endurance.

Athletes training for a specific goal, however, usually train for muscle endurance in a specific way. For repetitive-type sports such as running and swimming, where the movements are cyclic, the overall load need not be high. The repetitions involved are generally higher – between 20 and 30 – against a relatively lighter load of between 30 and 60%1RM. Rest periods between exercises would be up to two minutes.

For endurance sports such as rugby, hockey and American football, you would train differently. In terms of muscle endurance, you would exercise with higher loads. The movements in these sports are not as repetitive as in the cyclic sports, and they use the whole body in a variety of explosive movements. You would train between 60 and 80%1RM, performing between 8 and 20 explosive repetitions, and resting two to five minutes between sets.

The general programme does not focus on specific muscle endurance for specific sport types and is a guideline only. For muscle endurance, you need to perform high repetitions at relatively low resistances and, depending on the duration of the set, with relatively short rest periods. This programme has an upper-body lower-body split. A total-body approach can be equally effective.

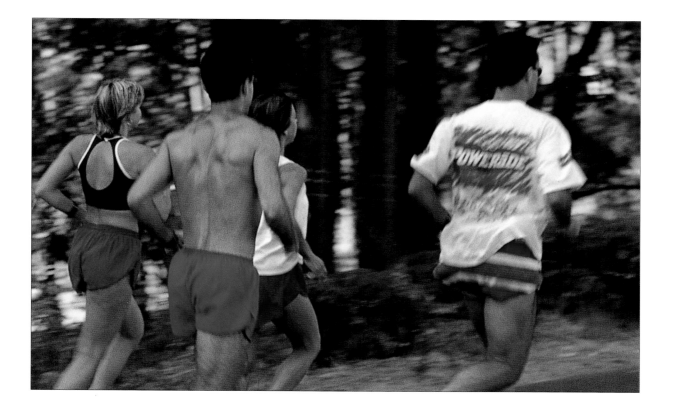

AN EXAMPLE OF A PROGRAMME FOR DEVELOPING MUSCLE ENDURANCE

Monday and Thursday – lower body

No.	Exercise	Load (%1RM)	Sets	Reps	Rest
1	Warm-up on stationary bicycle or treadmill, and stretch (±12–15min)	N/A	N/A	N/A	1–2min
2	Back squat	60–70%	3	15–20	60sec
3	Forward lunge	60–70%	3	15–20 per leg	60sec
4	Deadlift (bent-leg)	60–70%	3	15–20	60sec
5	Reverse crunch	N/A	3	15–20	30sec
6	Seated leg press	60–70%	3	15–20	60sec
7	Machine leg extension	60–70%	2	15–20	30sec
8	Prone leg curl	60–70%	2	15–20	30sec
9	Lying cross-overs	N/A	2	15–20	30sec
10	Standing calf raise	60–70%	3	15–20	30sec
11	Seated calf raise	60–70%	3	15–20	30sec
12	Cool-down on stationary bicycle or treadmill (±5–10min)	N/A	N/A	N/A	N/A

Comments: After the warm-up, perform all the sets for each exercise, from 2 to 11, before moving on to the cool-down.

Tuesday and Friday – upper body

No.	Exercise	Load (%1RM)	Sets	Reps	Rest
1	Warm-up on stationary bicycle or treadmill, and stretch (±12–15min)	N/A	N/A	N/A	1–2min
2	Incline bench press	60–70%	3	15–20	60sec
3	Bent-over row	60–70%	3	15–20	60sec
4	Incline sit-up	N/A	3	20–30	30sec
5	Behind-the-neck press	60–70%	3	15–20	60sec
6	Lat pulldowns	60–70%	3	15–20	60sec
7	Side raise	N/A	2	15–20 each side	30sec
8	Supine flye	60–70%	2	15–20	30sec
9	Bent-over cable lateral	60–70%	2	15–20	30sec
10	Shoulder shrug	60–70%	2	15–20	30sec
11	French press	60–70%	2	15–20	30sec
12	Concentration curl	60–70%	2	15–20	30sec
13	Cool-down on stationary bicycle or treadmill (±5–10min)	N/A	N/A	N/A	N/A

Comments: After the warm-up, perform all the sets for each exercise, from 2 to 12, before moving on to the cool-down.

Muscle toning

Increasing muscle tone involves firming up unused muscles. Any form of resistance training should achieve this goal. People wanting to be firm often worry that they will put on weight and become muscle-bound. For this reason, the variables in muscle-toning programmes are adapted to limit the amount of muscle mass accrued. Another outcome linked to muscle tone programmes is increased muscle definition. For more definition, you need to increase the number of sets per exercise, a common practice among bodybuilders before a competition.

For improved muscle tone, you need to use high repetitions – 12 to 15 repetitions per exercise – and medium loads of between 50 and 75%1RM, with a varying rest period between sets of between 30 seconds and two minutes, depending on the load and exercise.

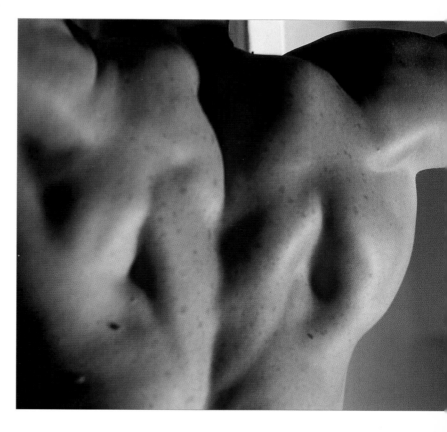

AN EXAMPLE OF A PROGRAMME FOR DEVELOPING MUSCLE TONE

No.	Exercise	Load (%1RM)	Sets	Reps	Rest
1	Warm-up on stationary bicycle or treadmill, and stretch (±12–15min)	N/A	N/A	N/A	1–2min
2	Flat bench press	60–70%	3	12–15	60sec
3	Bent-over barbell row	60–70%	3	12–15	60sec
4	Behind-the-neck press	60–70%	3	12–15	60sec
5	Incline flye	60–70%	2	12–15	30sec
6	Reverse flye	60–70%	2	12–15	30sec
7	Crane lunge	60–70%	3	12–15 per leg	60sec
8	Machine leg extensions	60–70%	2	12–15	30sec
9	Prone leg curls	60–70%	2	12–15	30sec
10	Reverse crunch	N/A	3	15–20	30sec
11	Seated calf raise	60–70%	3	15–20	30sec
12	Cool-down on stationary bicycle or treadmill (±5–10min)	N/A	N/A	N/A	N/A

Comments: After the warm-up, perform all the sets for each exercise, from 2 to 11, before moving on to the cool-down. Perform this workout two to three times a week.

Hypertrophy

For hypertrophy (muscle growth) you need to train individual muscles and muscle groups in high-volume workouts. For this type of programme to be effective, you need a lot of discipline, focus and, most importantly, time. You also need to follow an appropriate diet. Sports nutritionists may be more sympathetic to your needs than a dietician, whose interests are more general.

Such a programme starts with a general one-day, total-body workout and progresses to a two-day upper-body, lower-body split programme. The more advanced three-day, defined muscle-group split programme targets specific body parts or muscle groups with multiple sets and exercises on specified days. As the volume and load of this type of training is high, it is good practice to vary your exercise programme every six to eight weeks, otherwise you could stagnate and burn out.

For hypertrophy to be successful, you need to train at 70 to 85%1RM with 6 to 12 repetitions a set, and a rest period ranging from 30 to 90 seconds between exercises, depending on the load used. The short rest periods allow your muscle groups to recover just enough each time to enable you to perform the subsequent set. If you find you cannot perform them, your load may need to be adjusted to accommodate this.

The super-set is another training system frequently used in hypertrophy programmes and involves two exercises performed in succession, without rest. There are variations of super-sets, such as when an upper-body exercise is followed by a lower-body exercise; a pushing exercise is followed by a pulling exercise; an agonist exercise (for instance, involving the biceps) is followed by an antagonist exercise (involving the triceps); and two exercises are performed in succession involving the same muscle group. An example of the latter variation would be performing a bench press and following it immediately by a dumbbell French press. This example increases the overload on the triceps, as they are secondary muscles in the bench press and primary muscles in the French press.

These overloads result in a post-exercise increase in growth hormone (in both genders) and testosterone (in males), which stimulate muscle growth.

You should include aerobic activities every now and then to maintain general fitness and to limit your increase in body fat. This is because you will need to eat more to increase your energy intake, with the result that you run the risk of picking up a kilogram or two of fat together with muscle. Normally, you finish off a hypertrophy cycle by 'cutting' (*see glossary p122*) the muscles (through high repetitions and multiple sets) to increase muscle definition.

BEGINNER'S PROGRAMME

A programme for hypertrophy needs to focus on high-volume workouts involving all muscle groups at a relatively high intensity. Caution: it is important to listen to your body in order to avoid injury and burn-out.

INTERMEDIATE PROGRAMME

An intermediate programme incorporates an upper-body lower-body split programme. This is not the only way of

DIFFERENT SPLIT-PROGRAMME EXAMPLES

	Monday	Tuesday	Wednesday	Thursday	Friday	Saturday	Sunday
Total body	All major body parts	Rest	All major body parts	Rest	All major body parts	Rest	Rest
2-day split	Upper body	Lower body	Rest	Upper body	Lower body	Rest	Rest
3-day split	Chest and biceps	Upper back, shoulders and triceps	Lower back and legs	Chest and biceps	Upper back, shoulders and triceps	Lower back and legs	Rest

progressing, but I have found this to be an effective method. Remember to consult a sports nutritionist or dietician.

ADVANCED PROGRAMME

This is only for serious trainers who wish to gain significant muscle mass. Do not skip the earlier programmes. Remember that you need to eat right, train correctly and listen to your body.

Strength

Maximal strength is defined, in weight training circles, as the maximum weight a person can lift only once and correctly. Functional strength, however, is a basic necessity for everyday living. You do not need to lift

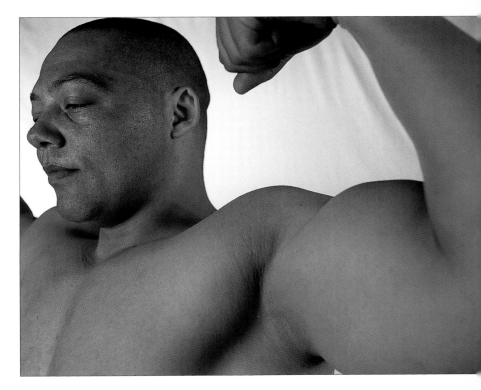

AN EXAMPLE OF A BEGINNER'S HYPERTROPHY PROGRAMME

No.	Exercise	Load (%1RM)	Sets	Reps	Rest	No.	Exercise	Load (%1RM)	Sets	Reps	Rest
1	Warm-up on stationary bicycle or treadmill, and stretch (±12–15min)	N/A	N/A	N/A	1–2min	9	Hip-adductor machine	70–75%	2	10	30sec
						10	Rowing torso	70–75%	2	10–12	30sec
2	Incline dumbbell bench press	70–75%	2–3	10–12	60sec	11	Incline sit-up	N/A	2	30–50	30sec
						12	Prone back extension	N/A	2	20–30	30sec
3	Back squat	70–75%	2–3	12–15	60sec	13	One-arm dumbbell press	70–75%	2	10–12	30sec
4	Supine flye	70–75%	2–3	10–12	30sec						
5	Crane lunge	70–75%	2–3	10 per leg	60sec	14	Donkey calf raise	N/A	2	20–30	30sec
6	Behind-the-neck press	70–75%	2–3	10–12	60sec	15	Alternated dumbbell curl	70–75%	2	10–12	30sec
7	Hip-abductor machine	70–75%	2	10	30sec	16	Seated calf raise	70–75%	2	15–20	30sec
8	Wide-grip chin-up	N/A	2–3	6–8	30sec	17	Cool-down on stationary bicycle or treadmill (±5–10min)	N/A	N/A	N/A	N/A

Comments: After the warm-up, perform all the sets for each exercise, from 2 to 16, before moving on to the cool-down. Perform this workout two to three times a week on alternate days.

AN EXAMPLE OF AN INTERMEDIATE HYPERTROPHY PROGRAMME

Monday and Thursday – lower body; Tuesday and Friday – upper body

This table shows only the Tuesday and Friday – upper body – routine

No.	Exercise	Load (%1RM)	Sets	Reps	Rest	No.	Exercise	Load (%1RM)	Sets	Reps	Rest
1	Warm-up on stationary bicycle or treadmill, and stretch (±12–15min)	N/A	N/A	N/A	1–2min	6	Military press	75–80%	4–5	8–10	90sec
						7	Lateral raise	75–80%	3–4	8–10	60sec
						8	French press	75–80%	3–4	8–10	60sec
2	Flat bench press	75–80%	4–5	8–10	90sec	9	Concentration curl	75–80%	3–4	8–10	60sec
3	Bent-over barbell-row	75–80%	4–5	8–10	90sec	10	Barbell wrist curl	N/A	3–4	12–15	30sec
4	Decline bench press	75–80%	4–5	8–10	90sec	11	Twist crunch	N/A	3	20–30	30sec
5	Lat pulldown	75–80%	4–5	8–10	60sec	12	Cool-down on stationary bicycle or treadmill (±5–10min)	N/A	N/A	N/A	N/A

Comments: After the warm-up, perform all the sets for each exercise, from 2 to 11, before moving on to the cool-down.
Additional comments: The lower-body training split follows the same approach as the upper-body routine above.

AN EXAMPLE OF AN ADVANCED HYPERTROPHY PROGRAMME

Monday and Thursday – chest, shoulders, triceps; Tuesday and Friday – lower body; Wednesday and Saturday – back, trapezius and biceps

This table shows only the Monday and Thursday – chest, shoulders, triceps – routine

No.	Exercise	Load (%1RM)	Sets	Reps	Rest	No.	Exercise	Load (%1RM)	Sets	Reps	Rest
1	Warm-up on stationary bicycle or treadmill, and stretch (±12–15min)	N/A	N/A	N/A	1–2min	8	Rowing torso	70–80%	4	8–12	60sec
						9	Narrow-grip bench press	70–80%	4	8–12	60sec
2	Incline dumbbell bench press	75–85%	5	6–10	90sec	10	Bench dip	N/A	4	20–30	60sec
3	Flat bench press	75–85%	5	6–10	90sec	11	Dumbbell kickback	70–80%	4	8–12	60sec
4	Dumbbell overhead press	75–85%	5	6–10	90sec	12	Knee-tuck	N/A	1	50	30sec
5	Straight-arm pullover	70–80%	4	8–12	60sec	13	Twist crunch	N/A	1	20–30	30sec
6	Lateral raise	70–80%	4	8–12	60sec	14	Cool-down on stationary bicycle or treadmill (±5–10min)	N/A	N/A	N/A	N/A
7	Machine flye	70–80%	4	8–12	60sec						

Comments:: After the warm-up, perform all the sets for each exercise, from 2 to 13, before moving on to the cool-down.
Additional comments: The other two training splits follow the same general approach as the Monday and Thursday routine above.

maximal weights to increase your functional strength. Any form of resistance training will improve it – even 30 to 80%1RM will increase your strength substantially. However, 80 to 100%1RM seems to be the most effective. Many people want to get stronger without significantly increasing muscle mass. When lifting heavy weights this is inevitable, but you can limit it by decreasing repetitions and increasing rest periods.

For improving strength, you need to perform one to eight repetitions in the 80 to 100%1RM range and rest two to eight minutes, depending on the load. Sufficient recovery allows your muscles to train optimally within each set of every exercise, thereby improving the rate at which your strength improves.

The Pyramid system can also be used for developing strength and involves progressively increasing weights while reducing the number of repetitions. For instance, a person on an intermediate strength-training programme using loads of 85 to 95%1RM will perform the first set (excluding warm-up sets) at 85%1RM for six repetitions; the following set at 90%1RM for four repetitions and the final set at 95%1RM for two repetitions. A variation of this is the Oxford system, which adopts the reverse order, starting with heavy weights and progressing to lighter ones: 95%1RM for two repetitions; 90%1RM for four repetitions and 85%1RM for six repetitions. There is also a combination of the Pyramid and Oxford systems: 85%1RM for six repetitions; 90%1RM for four repetitions; 95%1RM for two repetitions; 90%1RM for four repetitions and 85%1RM for six repetitions.

BEGINNER'S PROGRAMME

A strength-training programme is similar to the hypertrophy regimen, except that you perform fewer exercises per muscle group to develop functional strength. The load on the muscles is heavy so you should be careful.

INTERMEDIATE PROGRAMME

This intermediate training programme shifts towards an upper-body, lower-body split.

ADVANCED PROGRAMME

This programme is only for serious strength trainers. The format can also be used by people with less time, training three days a week on Mondays, Wednesdays and Fridays, but it would be less effective.

AN EXAMPLE OF A BEGINNERS' STRENGTH PROGRAMME

No.	Exercise	Load (%1RM)	Sets	Reps	Rest
1	Warm-up on stationary bicycle or treadmill, and stretch (±12–15min)	N/A	N/A	N/A	1–2min
2	Back squat	80–85%	3–4	8–10	2min
3	Incline bench press	80–85%	3–4	6–8	2min
4	Deadlift	80–85%	3–4	8–10	2min
5	Lat pulldown	75–85%	2–3	6–10	90sec

No.	Exercise	Load (%1RM)	Sets	Reps	Rest
6	Reverse flye	70–80%	2–3	8–12	60sec
7	One-arm dumb-bell press	70–80%	2–3	8–12	60sec
8	Concentration curl	70–80%	2–3	8–12	60sec
9	Hanging leg-raise	N/A	2	15–20	30sec
10	Twist crunch	N/A	2 each side	15–20	30sec
11	Cool-down on stationary bicycle or treadmill (±5–10min)	N/A	N/A	N/A	N/A

Comments: Do this workout three times a week on alternate days. Work on a heavy-light-medium day system: on the heavy day use the prescribed loads, on the light day loads of 80% of the first day's load and on the medium day 90%.

AN EXAMPLE OF AN INTERMEDIATE STRENGTH PROGRAMME

Monday and Thursday – lower body; Tuesday and Friday – upper body

This table shows only the Monday and Thursday – lower body – routine

No.	Exercise	Load (%1RM)	Sets	Reps	Rest	No.	Exercise	Load (%1RM)	Sets	Reps	Rest
1	Warm-up on stationary bicycle or treadmill, and stretch (±12–15min)	N/A	N/A	N/A	1–2min	6	Leg extension	70–80%	4	8–12	60sec
						7	Prone leg curl	70–80%	4	8–12	60sec
						8	Donkey calf raise	N/A	6	20–30	60sec
2	Back squat	80–95%	5	2–8	3min	9	Twist crunch	N/A	2 each side	15–20	30sec
3	Incline leg press	80–95%	5	2–8	3min						
4	Deadlift (bent leg)	80–95%	5	2–8	3min	10	Cool-down on stationary bicycle or treadmill (±5–10min)	N/A	N/A	N/A	N/A
5	Hanging leg-raise	N/A	2	20–25	30sec						

Comments: After the warm-up, perform all the sets for each exercise, from 2 to 9, before moving on to the cool-down. On the second day, do these exercises at 90% of load used on day one.

Additional comments: The upper body training split follows the same approach as the lower body routine above.

AN EXAMPLE OF AN ADVANCED STRENGTH PROGRAMME

Monday and Thursday – chest and biceps; Tuesday and Friday – lower body;
Wednesday and Saturday – upper back, shoulders and triceps

This table shows only the Monday and Thursday – chest and biceps – routine

No.	Exercise	Load (%1RM)	Sets	Reps	Rest	No.	Exercise	Load (%1RM)	Sets	Reps	Rest
1	Warm-up on stationary bicycle or treadmill, and stretch (±12–15min)	N/A	N/A	N/A	1–2min	6	Standing barbell curl	75–80%	3	8–10	60sec
						7	Concentration curl	75–80%	3	8–10	60sec
2	Flat bench press	85–95%	5	2–6	3–5min	8	Hammer curl	75–80%	3	8–10	60sec
3	Decline bench press	85–95%	5	2–6	3–5min	9	Machine crunch	70–80%	2	Max reps	30sec
4	Straight-arm pullover	80–85%	4	6–8	3min	10	Twisting crunch	N/A	2 each side	15–20	30sec
5	Machine flye	80–85%	4	6–8	3min	11	Cool-down on stationary bicycle or treadmill (±5–10min)	N/A	N/A	N/A	N/A

Comments: After the warm-up, perform all the sets for each exercise, from 2 to 10, before moving on to the cool-down. On the second day of the cycle, perform the exercises at 90% of the load used on the first day.

Additional comments: The other two training splits follow the same approach as the Monday and Thursday routine above.

Power

Power is defined as the amount of work performed over a time period. Work is the amount of force applied over a distance. In any exercise your range of motion remains pretty much fixed because the distance you cover during an exercise does not change much. So, the main factors to consider when power training are the loads lifted and the time spent lifting them. To increase power, you either have to increase your load or decrease the time period in which you are lifting the load by lifting the weights faster. However, if you increase the load too much, your speed of movement will be decreased and your power reduced, so you need to find a balance.

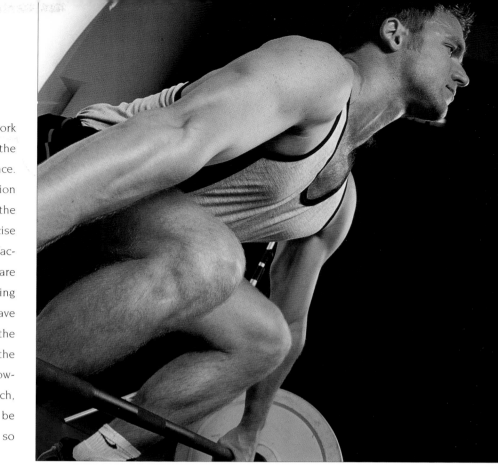

AN EXAMPLE OF A POWER-TRAINING PROGRAMME

Monday						Tuesday					
No.	Exercise	Load (%1RM)	Sets	Reps	Rest	No.	Exercise	Load (%1RM)	Sets	Reps	Rest
1	Warm-up on stationary bicycle or treadmill, and stretch (±12–15min)	N/A	N/A	N/A	1–2min	1	Warm-up on stationary bicycle or treadmill, and stretch (±12–15min)	N/A	N/A	N/A	1–2min
2	Clean-and-jerk	60–70%	5	2–5	4–5min	2	Hang snatch	50–60%	5	2–5	3min
3	Back squat	90%	5	4	3min	3	Rebound bench throw	30–40%	5	2–5	3min
4	Hang pull (snatch-grip)	60–70%	5	2–5	4–5min	4	Front raise	80%	3	8	90sec
5	Good morning (bent-leg)	80%	4	8	90sec	5	Cool-down on stationary bicycle or treadmill (±5–10min)	N/A	N/A	N/A	N/A
6	Cool-down on stationary bicycle or treadmill (±5–10min)	N/A	N/A	N/A	N/A						

Comments: After the warm-up, perform all the sets for each exercise, from 2 to 5, before moving on to the cool-down.

Comments: After the warm-up, perform all the sets for each exercise, from 2 to 4, before moving on to the cool-down..

		Thursday						Friday			
No.	Exercise	Load (%1RM)	Sets	Reps	Rest	No.	Exercise	Load (%1RM)	Sets	Reps	Rest
1	Warm-up on stationary bicycle or treadmill, and stretch (±12–15min)	N/A	N/A	N/A	1–2min	1	Warm-up on stationary bicycle or treadmill, and stretch (±12–15min)	N/A	N/A	N/A	1–2min
2	Hang clean	50–60%	5	2–5	3min	2	Power snatch	60–70%	5	2–5	4–5min
3	Push-jerk	50–60%	5	2–5	3min	3	Reverse lunge	40–50%	5	2–5	4–5min
4	Front squat	80%	5	6	3min	4	Incline bench press	90%	5	4	3min
5	Deadlift (bent-leg)	80%	5	6	3min	5	Cool-down on stationary bicycle or treadmill (±5–10min)	N/A	N/A	N/A	N/A
6	Reverse crunch	N/A	2	20–30	30sec						
7	Seated cable-row	80–85%	3	6	90sec						
8	One-arm dumbbell-press	70–80%	2	8	60sec						
9	Cool-down on stationary bicycle or treadmill (±5–10min)	N/A	N/A	N/A	N/A						

Comments: After the warm-up, perform all the sets for each exercise, from 2 to 8, before moving on to the cool-down.

Comments: After the warm-up, perform all the sets for each exercise, from 2 to 4, before moving on to the cool-down.

For optimal power development, your lifts should be performed explosively using loads of between 30 and 40%1RM. This is ideal for weighted plyometric exercises such as bench throws and jump squats, and single-joint exercises such as dumbbell lateral raises. Unfortunately, for most multijoint and total-body power exercises, these weights are too light and too much time is spent on slowing them down towards the end of a movement rather than on accelerating them, which is the primary goal of these exercises. The muscle groups are therefore not overloaded enough to develop functional power. Hence, in explosive lifts, loads ranging from 50 to 90%1RM are recommended. Olympic lifts and their variants, as well as resistive plyometric exercises, are mainly used to develop power. Traditional plyometric exercises, performed outside the gym, are also used to develop functional power and strength attributes that are partic-ularly beneficial for sportsmen and women. However, this is a fascinating study on its own and could be the subject for another book.

Power exercises should not be attempted by everyone. You need an adequate strength base, and you should be well schooled in the techniques beforehand.

All power exercises should be performed at the beginning of a training session and sufficient rest should be taken between sets and exercises. This is usually two to eight minutes, depending on the load used. The number of repetitions per set is usually between one and six, irrespective of the load.

If you have not been taught how to execute these exercises properly or do not yet have the requisite muscle conditioning, you should not attempt this programme as the risk of injury will be high. Depending on your training goals, these programmes can also differ significantly.

Summary

These programme templates are brief examples of how resistance-training exercises can be manipulated to achieve various goals. All sets exclude warm-ups. These samples do not cater for competitive sportsmen and women and their seasonal fluctuations and training schedules – the volume of their training would be significantly different and their training would be more specific.

The templates for weight loss and muscle tone cater for people who have undergone medical and physical fitness screening and who have already undertaken preconditioning classes such as cliniband, pezzi-ball or body-mass exercises. The remaining routine workouts are for those who have also undergone a basic conditioning programme. All these templates can be adapted to individual needs and modified to allow for time constraints.

Participants will respond differently to each training programme and fitness professionals can prescribe programmes accordingly. Before proceeding to a new level, whether intermediate or advanced, you should undergo a general assessment of your cardiovascular fitness, muscle strength and body composition for optimal programme structuring and load determination. This should in any case be done on a regular basis to monitor the effectiveness of your training programme and to guide the fitness professional to make adjustments.

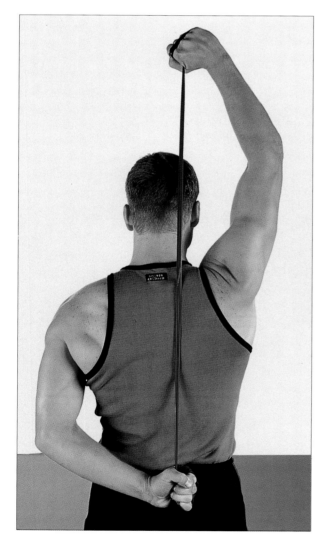

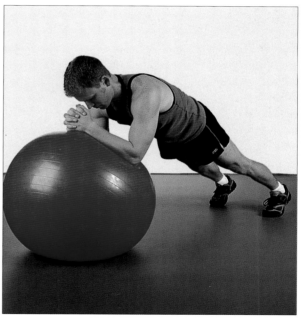

Above: Pezzi-ball exercises are excellent for training the core stabilizing muscles such as the transversus abdominus, multifidus, and quadratus lumborum. These can improve balance and muscular coordination, decrease the prevalence of injuries and lead to more efficient muscle power.

Left: Theraband or surgical tubing can contribute to muscle conditioning, although they do not have the same range of effectiveness as weight training. For people who are undergoing rehabilitation, are aged and/or very unfit, this can be a beneficial and reasonably inexpensive training tool.

Glossary

1 RM: One-repetition maximum: the maximum load that an individual can correctly lift only once through a complete range of motion in a specific exercise. It is used for prescribing the amount of weight to be used.

Abduction: Any movement of a limb away from the centreline of the body such as lifting a straight arm laterally from one's side.

Abs: The abdominal (stomach) muscles.

Adduction: Any movement of a limb towards the centreline of the body such as pulling a straight arm towards one's side.

Agonist: The primary muscle that contracts to create a specific movement, for instance the bicep in a bicep curl.

Air displacement plethysmography: A technique of calculating body density and percentage body-fat. A person sits in a closed chamber while computerized pressure sensors measure the amount of air displaced by the individual's body.

Anatomical position: (Illustration right) The neutral standing position from which all movements are described. The movement descriptions of each joint are in reference to their anatomical positions.

Antagonist: The primary muscle that opposes a specific movement, for instance, the tricep in a bicep curl.

Anterior: The front side.

Barbell: The long metal bar on which weights are placed. Used for free-weight training. A variation of the standard barbell is the Olympic bar that weighs about 20kg (44 lb) and has rotating sleeves that allow for wrist rotation.

Bioelectrical impedance: A method of measuring body composition, based on the premise that muscle, bone and lean tissue are better electrical conductors than body fat, mainly due to a higher water content. A low electrical current is passed through the body. The resistance is measured and used in the calculation.

Abduction

Adduction

Frontal plane   Sagittal plane

Transverse plane

Burn-out: A condition experienced by athletes and weight trainers when they are overtrained or severely fatigued. Unchecked, it can lead to chronic illness and fatigue.

Collars and locks: Used to secure weights onto barbells and dumbbells. The weights are slid along the bar until they are pressed against the collar. The lock is slid along the bar until pressed against the weights, where it is tightened in place. This prevents the weights from slipping off the barbells and dumbbell bars during training.

Cutting: Reducing body fat and increasing muscle definition by incorporating higher repetitions, more sets and smaller loads used during weight training.

Delts: The deltoid or shoulder muscles.

Dual-energy X-ray absorptiometry (DEXA): A technique to determine total body fat and lean-tissue mass, using an X-ray scan and computer software to reconstruct and image underlying tissue. It is a noninvasive radiological projection technique, which differentiates directly between various tissue densities.

Dumbbells: These are free weights, similar to the standard barbell, but significantly smaller and shorter.

Energy-system training: Training focused on manipulating loads, repetitions, rest periods and sets in order to tax an energy system particular to a sport type.

Extension: Extending a joint, or opening the angle between two bones, in the sagittal plane so that they diverge (angle increases).

External rotation: The outward or lateral rotation of a joint within the transverse plane of the body. The movement is towards the back of the body.

Flexion: Flexing a joint or closing the angle between two bones in the sagittal plane; the two bones approach each other.

Frontal plane: The body's vertical division into a front and back half. Movements in the frontal plane are lateral and conducted away and towards the body's centreline, namely side-to-side or left-to-right (*see abduction and adduction*).

Glutes: The gluteus or buttock muscles.

Hammies: The hamstrings or back-thigh muscle group.

Hydrostatic (underwater) weighing: A technique using body density to calculate body composition, based on Archimedes' principle that the volume of an object is proportional to its loss of weight when measured in water. A person is strapped in a chair and submerged while expelling all air from the lungs. Because fat is less dense than water, it contributes to the individual's buoyancy. Body density and percentage body fat are calculated from the person's underwater weight. The less weight, the more body fat.

Hyperextension: The extension of a joint beyond the anatomical position.

Inferior: To be below, lower or at the bottom.

Infrared scanning: A technique for estimating percentage body fat, called near-infrared spectroscopy. An infrared sensor is pressed against the skin, projecting an infrared beam and measuring the absorption of the emission. Body fat absorbs the light and lean tissue reflects it, therefore the more body fat, the greater the absorption of light.

Internal rotation: The inward or medial rotation of a joint within the transverse plane of the body. Movement is directed towards the anterior surface or front of the body.

Lats: The latissimus dorsi or upper-back muscles.

Load/intensity: The weight to be used in kilograms or pounds.

Maximal: As close to a maximum unit reading as possible.

Multijoint: Actively involving more than one joint.

Muscle tone: A term referring to firm muscles.

Olympic lifts: Athletic-type, explosive exercises using an Olympic bar such as in the clean-and-jerk and the snatch.

Overload: Training harder than what one is used to.

Pecs: The pectoralis or chest muscles.

Posterior: Located behind a part or toward the rear of the body.

Primary movement: The main movement around a specific joint.

Pronation: The internal rotation of the foot or forearm.

Quads: The quadricep muscle group.

ROM: Range of motion.

Reps: (Repetitions) Number of times a movement is done.

Rest: Time rested between sets and exercises.

RM: (Repetition maximum) In the case of 12RM, for example, a load that only allows 12 repetitions.

Sagittal plane: A division that separates the body into a left and right half. Movements in the sagittal plane are in the forward-backward direction (see flexion and extension).

Set: Group of repetitions separated by a rest period.

Spotting: External support provided to prevent injury and to assist training persons when they reach muscle failure.

Submaximal: Less than the maximum load you can lift.

Superior: Above, on top of, or upper.

Supination: The external rotation of the foot or forearm.

Supramaximal: More than the maximum load you can lift.

Transverse plane: The division separating the body into an upper and lower half. Movements are in the horizontal direction or parallel to the ground (see internal and external rotation).

Ultrasonographic studies: Studies using computer-captured ultrasonic measurements.

Volume: Amount of work done in a training session, calculated as the sum of the products of the respective weights, repetitions and sets undertaken in that session. The volume of work is also sometimes measured as the multiplication of the sets and repetitions.

Dumbbells
Locks
Collar
Olympic Bar
Standard Bar
EZ-bar

Index

Useful Information

Equipment

Alphafitness

www.alphafitnessequipment.com

Apexfit www.apexfit.com/catalog

Back Health www.backhealth.com

Bowflex www.bowflex.com

Fitness 1st www.fitness1st.com

HealthFX America

www.healthfxamerica.com

Power Systems

www.power-systems.com

Sports Strength www.sportstrength.com

Tuffstuff www.tuffstuff.net

Zest Manufacturing (Pty) Ltd

www.zestfitness.com

Organizations

INTERNATIONAL ORGANIZATIONS

International Natural Bodybuilding

Association

www.naturalbodybuilding.com

The International Federation of

Bodybuilders

www.getbig.com/info/ifbb.htm

World Federation of Natural Athletes

www.wfna.net

World Fitness Federation

www.worldfitnessfederation.com

World Natural Bodybuilding

Federation (WABBA) www.wnbf.net

World Natural Sports Organization

www.worldnaturalsports.com

UNITED KINGDOM

British Natural Bodybuilding

Association www.bnbf.co.uk

National Amateur Bodybuilding

Association (NABBA) www.nabba.com

Association of Natural Bodybuilders

UK see 'Links' 'Great Britain' at

www.ocbbodybuilding.com

AUSTRALIA

Australasian Natural Bodybuilding

(ANB) www.anb.com.au

Natural Bodybuilding Inc.

www.nbibodybuilding.com

UNITED STATES

American College of Sports Medicine

www.acsm.org

American Council on Exercise

www.acefitness.org

International Sport Science

Association (ISSA)

www.issaonline.com

National Strength and Conditioning

Association (NSCA) www.nsca-lift.org

The Amateur Athletic Union

www.aausports.org

The National Physique Committee

www.getbig.com

United Natural Bodybuilding

Association www.unbainc.com

United States Natural Bodybuilding

Association (USNBA)

www.tpgonline.us

Natural Bodybuilding Publications

MAGAZINES

Flex www.Flexonline.com

Gen-Mag www.gen-mag.com

Health & Fitness www.Hfonline.co.uk

Men's Fitness Available from

www.amazon.com

Ms Fitness www.msfitness.com

Muscle & Fitness Available from

www.amazon.com

Muscle & Fitness Hers

www.muscleandfitnesshers.com

Natural Muscle www.naturalmuscle.net

Planet Muscle www.planetmuscle.com

Further reading

SUPPLEMENTARY TRAINING

Body Shaping With Free Weights:
Easy Routines for Your Home
Workout *Stephenie Karony,*
Anthony L. Ranken

Sports Illustrated Training with Weights:
The Athlete's Free-Weight Guide
Robert B. Baker

SPORTS PSYCHOLOGY

Handbook of Sport Psychology
Robert N. Singer

The Mental Edge: Maximise Your Sports
Potential with the Mind/Body
Connection *Ken Baum, Richard Trubo*
(contributor), *Kenneth H. Baum,*
Karch Kiraly

NUTRITION

Complete Guide to Sports Nutrition
Monique Ryan

Nancy Clark's Sports Nutrition
Guidebook, 2nd edition *Nancy Clark*

Power Eating *Susan M. Kleiner, Maggie*
Greenwood-Robinson (Contributor)

Supplements for Strength-Power
Athletes *Jose Antonio, Jeffrey R. Stout*

The Bodybuilder's Nutrition Book
Franco Columbu, Lydia Fragomeni

Acknowledgements

Dedication

To my father Herc and mother Lucille; Chanté, Theo, Leon and Catherine;
and a special dedication to my uncle Boy, who passed away recently.

Author's Acknowledgements

Eugene Vogel and his staff from Eugene Fashions/Sports Clobber,
Cape Town, South Africa, for designing and sponsoring of the
outfits used for the photo-shoot.

The Wellness and Fitness Centre and the Discovery Health
High Performance Centre at the Sports Science Institute of South Africa,
for the use of their equipment and facilities.

The Claremont Virgin Active Gymnasium, Cape Town, South Africa
for the use of their equipment and facilities.

Catherine Harrison-Smith and Michele Boddington, who were available
at all times to bounce ideas off and painstakingly read through
my initial drafts. Their input was most appreciated.

Yolande Harley, Bridgette Ray, Ingrid Peens and Denzil van Heerden who
took time off their busy work schedules to model for the photo-shoot.

All the staff at New Holland Publishing (South Africa)
who were very supportive and helpful.